INTRODUCTION
TO QUANTUM
WELLNESS

ADDITIONAL RESOURCES:

Enjoy these reader resources at https://quantumhumandesign.com/quantum-wellness-book!

Experience the Masterclass Series: Watch our masterclass series videos and hear Dr. Karen deliver valuable information you can implement now.

Access Quantum Alignment System Professional Training: Explore our certification course if you'd like to add QAS to your current practice or for your personal transformation. As a special gift, apply code QASRESOURCE to save 20%!

EFT for Everyone Ebook: A quick primer for those new to Emotional Freedom Techniques.

Vitality Sound Frequency: A deeply relaxing sound frequency designed to help you calibrate your energy to a higher state of vitality.

Flower Essences from The Potion Lady: premium subtle body products developed exclusively to augment your journey through the Quantum Alignment System.

Quantum Alignment System Bibliography: A comprehensive list of research citations and recommended reading for diving deeper into the modalities found in QAS.

Other Books and Resources by Dr. Karen Curry Parker

Understanding Human Design

Human Design Workbook

Inside the Body of God

Introduction to Quantum Human Design™ 3rd Edition

The Quantum Human: The Evolution of Consciousness and the Solar Plexus Mutation in Human Design

LEARN MORE ABOUT QUANTUM HUMAN DESIGN:

HTTPS://QUANTUMHUMANDESIGN.COM

INTRODUCTION TO QUANTUM WELLNESS

INTEGRATING HUMAN DESIGN FOR OPTIMAL WELL-BEING

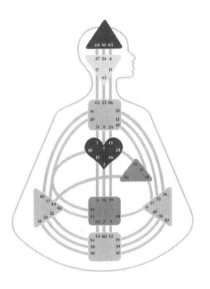

DR. KAREN CURRY PARKER

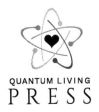

QUANTUM LIVING
PRESS

Published in the United States by Quantum Living Press in 2024

Introduction To Quantum Wellness: Integrating Human Design For Optimum Well-Being

The content of this book is for informational purposes only and is not intended to diagnose, treat, cure, or prevent any condition or disease. You understand that this book is not intended as a substitute for consultation with a licensed practitioner. Please consult with your own physician or healthcare specialist regarding the suggestions and recommendations made in this book. The use of this book implies your acceptance of this disclaimer.

Quantum Living Press
Quantum Alignment System, LLC

2112 Broadway St NE Ste 225, #305
Minneapolis, MN 55413

www.quantumhumandesign.com
www.freehumandesignchart.com
Email: support@quantumhumandesign.com

A Library of Congress Control Number has been requested and is pending.

ISBN (Paperback): 979-8-9910244-0-2

eISBN: 979-8-9910244-1-9

First Edition 2024

Books may be purchased for educational, business, or sales promotional use.

For bulk order requests and price schedule contact:

support@quantumhumandesign.com

DEDICATION

For Team Quantum and all the Cosmic Revolutionaries who are paving the way for a world of equitable, just, abundant, and sustainable peace.

TABLE OF CONTENTS

Introduction...3

Chapter 1: The "Quantum Mechanics" of How We Create 7

Chapter 2: An Integrated Approach to Optimal Wellness
and Well-Being...17

Chapter 3: Overview of QHD - Type/Strategy/Authority 27

Initiator / Manifestor... 30

Alchemist / Generator 39

Time Bender / Manifesting Generator 47

Orchestrator / Projector 55

Calibrator / Reflector...63

QAS Alignment Protocols:

Initiator / Manifestor..78

Alchemist / Generator 81

Time Bender / Manifesting Generator 84

Orchestrator / Projector 87

Calibrator / Reflector 91

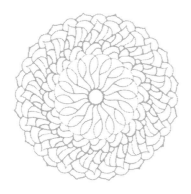

INTRODUCTION

Our bodies are malleable and responsive to many factors. Bodies react to stress, age, season, environment, diet, activity levels, ancestral lineage, and more. Creating optimal well-being in the body is dependent on countless factors. Each body, and every season of the body, will react to treatment in different ways. Even though we can often predict, to a certain degree, how the body will respond to treatments, treating the body as a unique phenomenon is essential when we focus on the variety of factors that create disease and stress in the body.

We are trained to see the body as a machine that heals through a formulaic approach. We often treat pain without exploring the underlying cause of the pain. When the pain resolves, we assume we are healed without dealing with the underlying cause. Without treating the underlying cause, the body is vulnerable to experiencing unending cycles of pain, disease, or chronic conditions.

Thirty years ago, when I first became a nurse, not many people were exploring the impact of emotions, personal narrative - even ancestral trauma - on pain and disease in the body. In recent years, physicians, Mount Sinai School of Medicine neuroscientist Dr. Rachel Yehuda, psychiatrist Bessel van der Kolk, author of *The Body Keeps the Score*, and renowned mental health expert and speaker Dr. Gabor Maté, we're now seeing the relationship between our personal and collective stories, and the health of the body.

Our emotional legacy is hidden, encoded in everything from gene expressions to everyday language. This legacy plays a far greater role in our emotional and physical health than has ever before been understood. As we grow up, we internalize the message that it's not okay, or safe, for us to be who we are. This chronic state of self-denial causes us to deplete our vital life-force energy as we try to safely keep our true selves hidden away.

Most of us have also learned to silence our body's wisdom and the messages our precious physical vehicle gives us. True healing requires reconnection with the body's wisdom and remembering how our body feels when something is right for us—or not.

When we are not connected to our body, it is forced to get our attention through physical pain and burnout. The body finds a way of letting us know we are wildly off course from our true path.

We can use the power of intentional storytelling to assess and, ultimately, transform the body and enhance optimal wellness and well-being. We can do this when we begin to see the body as a key element in a feedback loop of information that metaphorically reveals the root cause of pain and disease.

But before we can do this, we have to explore what story we are telling ourselves and the world about who we are. We have to remember what we once knew: how to interpret the messages our bodies are giving us.

This book is intended to introduce the Quantum Alignment System, an integrated system that incorporates Quantum Human Design, Energy Psychology techniques, Flower Essences, Healing Sound Frequencies, and intentional storytelling to help you get to the archetypal root of physical, mental, and spiritual pain.

This book is both a mini-workbook for personal discovery meant to introduce an integrated approach to using Quantum Human Design as an assessment tool and a way of helping your clients take control over their personal narrative to create greater physical, emotional, and spiritual well-being in their lives.

There is a correlation between the stories we tell the world (and ourselves) about who we are and what we experience in life. In this mini-ebook, you'll learn about the quantum physics and physiology of creativity and how your personal story influences what you create-

-even in your body. As you explore your personal narrative and its impact on your health and well-being, you'll gain powerful insights into how your body is giving you vital information to help you create optimal wellness.

This introductory book provides a cursory overview of how to integrate Quantum Human Design into your wellness practice and use it as a tool to help others.

Each chapter begins with a brief review of the major concepts essential to understanding the chapter's content. Each chapter builds on the next, and there are many new ideas in each chapter. Take your time and reflect on the review content before reading the next chapter to quickly integrate the new information.

You will need a copy of your Quantum Human Design chart to complete these exercises. You can get your personal Quantum Human Design chart at http:/www.freehumandesignchart.com.

Even if you have your Human Design chart, you'll want a copy of your chart that uses the Quantum Human Design language.

Everything you learn from this book is about stories and the correlation between your story and your well-being. The intention here is to optimize wellness and explore these correlations. Please use this information to augment your well-being. This information is not intended to replace a professional diagnosis or professional care.

Most of all, be gentle with yourself. You are here for a reason. You are on a journey of growth and expansion. Everything in your life has brought you to this place. Celebrate the sacredness of your journey and acknowledge how far you've come!

CHAPTER 1

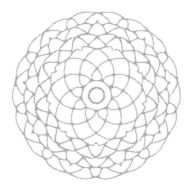

THE "QUANTUM MECHANICS" OF HOW WE CREATE

In a world that sometimes makes you feel like you're out of control, it's only natural you try to find meaning and a sense of power over what happens to you - including what happens to your body and your health. In recent years, the spiritual practice of manifesting has become part of popular jargon and practice. You might have tried manifesting using visualization, vision boards, or even affirmations to create something you want in your life.

Manifesting is often distilled down to the idea that your thoughts create your reality.

In other words, if you think it, it will come true. The better skilled you are at regulating what you think, the better you get at manifesting. While thoughts are certainly part of the creative process, most people who try manifesting by simply "thinking" something into being are left feeling frustrated.

For years, I taught a program called Prosperity Bootcamp. I created this course to help people learn how to get a better sense of control over the manifesting process in their lives. Mostly, I taught the class for myself because, at that time, I was struggling with my own manifesting, and I thought if I taught this process to others, it would keep me steeped in the information, so I could also see the results I hoped for.

Prosperity Bootcamp was filled with students who had followed the concept of "your thoughts create your reality" with great zest and very few results. Personally, I had variable results with my "manifesting," even though I was pretty consistent with my visualizing and affirming. Despite the fact I was using my mind with all my might to try to tackle my financial challenges and my relationship issues, it didn't seem to really be working very well for me.

At the time, I was a full-time single mom of four children. I was struggling to grow my business so I could create the resources to take care of my family. My dating life was miserable. I had a slew of relationships that reflected my own inner lack of value. There was very little time or energy left in my day for myself and my own self-renewal. I was living in survival mode, just trying to keep everything afloat.

One day, I found a lump in my breast. I was so terrified I ignored it for a few months until I couldn't risk denying the problem any longer. As a nurse and an energy healer, I knew I could visualize health and potentially improve the situation. I affirmed complete and total health on a daily basis, hoping the lump would go away, but it didn't. Finally, fearing my children would lose their mother, I eventually found the courage to go to the doctor and face the reality of a cancer diagnosis.

I kept my breast cancer a secret from everyone. I struggled through surgery alone, stoic, and self-reliant. Even though I faced pain, fear, and illness, I continued to take care of my family and focus on my work. I had no friends. I didn't want to burden my parents, who had already done so much for me. I didn't want to talk about my illness with my clients or online because I felt like my cancer was a manifestation of failure. My body clearly demonstrated I had no control over my thinking and, consequently, what I manifested.

After surgery, I was given Tamoxifen (hormonal therapy) to prevent recurrence. The Tamoxifen made my mood and my outlook on life extremely bleak. I struggled every day with deep depression, which is a common side-effect of Tamoxifen. The depression only served to deepen my sense of spiritual failure.

The quality of my life continued to decline. The stress from being ill, continuing to take care of my children, and the financial burdens that took a toll on my mind, body, and spirit seemed to never end. I couldn't figure out how, as a metaphysical teacher, a long-time mediator, and a person with affirmations plastered all over my house, I could be failing - in such a phenomenal way - to manifest perfect health. (Heck, at that point, I would have settled for manifesting feeling slightly BETTER!)

I was at my wit's end until one day, during meditation a voice in my head asked me how I would treat myself if I were my own client. This question stopped me cold. I realized if I was my own client, I would advise myself to start looking at my experience as a metaphor for my life. If my life was a story and my body was giving me vital information about my story, what was my body trying to tell me?

I sat quietly with this contemplation and became deeply aware that my body was crying out to be heard. As I listened and explored the messages my body had for me, I realized that breasts are a metaphor for nurturing. The manifestation of cancer in my breast held the story of my body and my life, crying out for self-care and rest. I needed succor, spiritual nourishment, and support to be receptive to love, nurturing, and more balance in my life. I realized that in plowing forward to be everything I needed to be for my family and for my business, coupled with the fear that if I failed, I'd be letting everyone else down, I had neglected myself.

This neglect led to my body crying out and begging me to stop and nurture myself.

For me, the first step was to stop taking Tamoxifen. (This was an incredibly personal decision, and if you're facing similar issues, please consult your medical team before making a similar choice.) I needed to reconnect with my natural emotional energy in order to recalibrate and begin the process of creating a better story for my life.

Slowly, I added self-care and nurturing into my daily life. It was a very steep learning curve as I soon discovered how deeply I had been conditioned by martyrdom. I reconnected with old memories of being praised for giving up what I wanted and needed for the sake of others. I realized I had internalized stories from the women in my family that lauded their sacrifices, turning them into saints who gave it all for their loved ones, regardless of the cost to their health and well-being. My own grandmother was praised for her patience and kindness when she accepted my grandfather's infidelity.

I eventually realized there was no merit in martyring myself, and I could create whatever life I wanted. In fact, I discovered I actually could do more for everyone, including myself, when I took care of myself first. I worked hard to rewrite our family narrative so my children would grow up with a mother who understood how to create healthy harmony in her life and who modeled self-care.

My strength returned. My body and I began a partnership to create my health. I listened to my body carefully and rested proactively with gusto - an entirely new way of living!

Obviously, the restoration of my health was my biggest takeaway, but I also learned something vital about the manifesting process.

You can think of all the good thoughts you want, but they won't manifest if your underlying story is incongruous with what you are trying to manifest. To truly create what you want, you have to tell a story about who and how you are. This story has to match how much you trust and believe you are worthy to receive what you really want.

My body taught me to value myself enough to take care of myself. I had to begin to believe I deserved rest, support, and nurturing in order to rewrite the story of all of my previous life experiences. I realized that nothing outside of me could devalue me: not my ex-husband, not my ancestral lineage, not my finances.

I learned if I wanted more money, better health, more free time, and the presence to truly be with my children, I had to have an underlying story that precluded all of these outcomes. Once I internalized this understanding, I began to heal my story, and my life's creations shifted dramatically.

THE PARTS OF THE MANIFESTING EQUATION

In order to manifest, you have to understand the different components of the manifesting process. The manifesting process isn't just about mindset and thinking. It's a powerful physiological process.

To truly take control of the manifestation process, you have to change the way you think, live more authentically, and reclaim sovereignty over your personal story. You literally have to change your body and cultivate a practice that keeps you aligned with your natural creative power.

Let's start by exploring the parts of the manifesting equation before you learn how to put all of these parts together to give you a formula for cultivating well-being and expansion, no matter what's happening in your life.

As you conceptualize all of these different parts of the manifesting equation, please remember most of these parts do not exist on the material plane.

You are learning to become a master of energy and reclaiming your power to transform this energy into form.

THE QUANTUM FIELD OF INFINITE POTENTIAL

Right now, as you read this, you are sitting in the middle of a field of information that contains every single potential for all of reality. It's not manifested yet. This field is pure potential and contains the energetic building blocks that make up any situation, opportunity, or thing you can dream of.

Your human brain can only imagine an infinitesimal portion of the potentials available in the cosmos.

This field of information is full of quantum particles that move at the speed of light (photons) and even faster than the speed of light (tachyons).

When quantum physicists first tried to explain and measure quantum particles, they soon discovered they could either measure the movement of a particle or the location of a particle, but never both at the same time. As soon as the scientist had an expectation about where a quantum particle could be located, the particle dropped out of movement into its expected material form. In other words, the particle behaved as expected.

Moving quantum particles represent potential. They aren't actually "manifested" yet on the material plane. Quantum particles that have "located" drop out of movement and exist on the material plane.

The meaning (expectation) we have about potentials determines how they drop out of movement and are made manifest on the material plane. The meanings you hold for the potentials of your life are determined by the second part of the manifesting equation, your Conditioning Field.

YOUR CONDITIONING FIELD

You have a field of information surrounding you that contains the entire history of who you are and all the things that have ever happened to you. This field of information includes all of your past experiences, emotions, and beliefs related to these experiences. It also includes memories stored in your body, including memories from your ancestral lineage.

Your Quantum Human Design - your unique energy blueprint - is also part of your conditioning field.

Living in a field of information that contains infinite potential is overwhelming and untenable for most people. You have unlimited choices for what you can create with your life. Your human body and mind can not process this much information without being completely overwhelmed and overloaded.

Your conditioning field essentially acts like a filter. It helps you "choose" which possibilities you're going to pluck out of the Quantum Field and manifest in your life.

Your conditioning field is programming what you create and experience in your life. Your personal narrative, the story you tell yourself and the world about who you are, is crafted from your conditioning field. This story sets the tone and direction for your life and has tremendous influence over what and how you manifest.

THE SUBTLE BODY

The Subtle Body is your aura, the natural energy field that surrounds your body. This energy field is a template holding together the energetic structure for what you are experiencing in your life right now.

If you've ever had any kind of energy "healing" such as Reiki or Healing Touch or used essential oils, the flower essences of homeopathy, these treatments work on the subtle body level.

A good intuitive medical empath or psychic can "look" at your subtle body energy field and "see" if you've been ill or you're about to be ill because they can see changes in your subtle body. They might even be able to see whether your "soulmate" or money is coming into your life because the changes in your physical reality exist in the subtle body first.

The Subtle Body is often a piece of the creation equation that is ignored. You accelerate and strengthen the creation process when you also work on the Subtle Body level.

To create real change, you have to start by changing the stories you hold in your conditioning field. You have to rethink, and rewrite, your old narrative. Reclaiming sovereignty over the events that have led to your current story. This means you have to change your mind, your

12

thinking, and the patterns in your body. You also have to shift the habits you've formed in response to your old story.

Even though inner change can be instant, it can sometimes take time for your body to catch up with the changes, especially if parts of your old story had elements you cultivated to protect you and help you feel safe.

When you first start changing your story, you're vulnerable. You've disrupted your old story. You can't go back to how things used to be - even though it's tempting. It's common to feel, as your new story is gaining strength, like you're sitting in a sort of void or a gap between your old story and your new story.

Sometimes, when you're in the void, old artifacts from your previous stories pop back up into your reality. An old boyfriend comes back. You get hit with an unexpected bill. You hang out with your old friends, and you start to doubt the new direction you're trying to take in your life.

It's easy to make changes to your story, start the inner deconditioning process, and immediately go out into the world and get reconditioned again. It's ironic that sometimes we're trying to decondition the exact environment where we were conditioned in the first place. It can feel like a test of sorts. This is the time when a lot of people give up and stop trying to create something different.

Bolstering the changes you make by adding subtle body therapies, such as flower essences, can strengthen your new story and help hold it in place until it integrates into your body. Subtle body therapies serve as a kind of band-aid or poultice, helping to hold the changes you desire in place until you can integrate them deeply into every layer of your being.

YOUR PHYSICAL REALITY

The last component of the manifesting process is finally experiencing your creative intention, and your story changes on the material plane. As you will learn in the next section, your physical reality is part of an elegant feedback loop that mirrors back to you the changes you've made in your story and your energy field. The more you decondition yourself, take back control of your story, and learn how to regulate your subtle body, the more your physical reality will be as you have imagined it. The better you get at this process, the more you learn to be in alignment with not only creating what you want, but influencing the timing of when what you want shows up!

Your physical reality is malleable, infinite, and never set in stone. One of the most important things you have to do to become a fully activated Creative, is to realize all of reality is a story that's been made manifest. If you don't like what you see around you, it's not locked or fixed. You have the power to choose how you're going to experience your world.

HOW IT WORKS

Now that you know the parts of the creative equation, let's put all the parts together so you can start to work with these parts to deliberately create what you want for your life.

Let's start with a simple exercise. You'll need a paper and a pen to get started.

Think of the word "money".

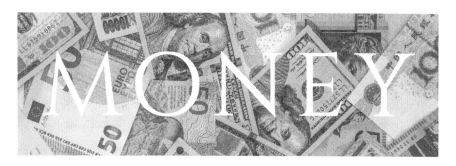

Write down every thought or feeling you experience when you think of the word "money."

When you're done, put your hand over your heart, take a nice long deep breath and bring your awareness back to this book.

Here's what happened as you completed this exercise.

As soon as your eyes saw the word "money," your brain produced a photon (light) storm. Photons flash through the nerve connections in your brain, causing your brain to produce chemicals called neurotransmitters.

Congratulations! You are so powerful you literally just transformed light into matter!

These neurotransmitters travel through your body and produce an emotional response. The emotional response you created matches your emotional programming - your conditioning - around your money story.

Let's say, for example, you have a fear that whenever you have money, you mismanage it, and you lose it all. Whenever you think about money, this part of your money "story" gets activated, and your body responds by creating neurotransmitters that stimulate emotions that match this story.

Emotional energy carries a frequency that is variable depending on which emotions are generated. High-frequency emotional energy calibrates your mind and body into a state of coherence. Coherence happens when the heart, mind, and emotions are in alignment and cooperation. When you are in a state of coherence, you experience ease, a sense of well-being, and greater creativity.

Low-frequency emotional energy, including stress, fear, anxiety, or despair, puts your body in a state of non-coherence. Your thoughts and emotions trigger a low-grade fight-or-flight response. Your body and mind prepare to run or take defensive action, and your brain shuts down your natural creative response, causing you to be more reactive instead of conscious and deliberate.

In addition to these emotional responses, your thoughts program your brain to look for evidence in your outer world that matches the story you're telling yourself. You are bombarded with thousands of bits of information a second. Your brain, which has beautifully evolved to be focused and attentive, can only process about 120 bits of information a second.

In order to not go on information overload, your brain is programmed to sort through all the data you're being bombarded with. It only processes the bits of information that are relevant to you. Your brain has a system called the Reticular Activating System (RAS) that programs which bits of data have meaning to you. The story you tell about yourself, and your life, programs the RAS to pay attention to the bits of information your brain is processing so you see the "evidence" of your story in your outer world. This reinforces the perceived "truth" of your story, causing you to potentially get stuck in old stories that don't actually help you create what you want and deserve in your life.

This is why the story you tell about yourself, including the way in which you interpret your Quantum Human Design chart, is such an essential part of what and how you create. Your story (including the meanings you give your Quantum Human Design) is simply a filter through which we see potentials, create expectations that cause these potentials to manifest on the material plane, and interpret them through the preprogramming of the RAS in your mind so your outer reality seemingly appears to mirror your inner world.

To transform your reality, you must reclaim sovereignty over your personal narrative and your inner world. If you are the source of the experience of reality in your life, you must first know who you are. If you are unhappy with the reality you are experiencing, to transform it, you have to change the story you tell about who you are.

CHAPTER 2

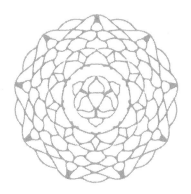

AN INTEGRATED APPROACH TO OPTIMAL WELLNESS AND WELL-BEING

REVIEW:

- The stories you tell the world (and yourself) about who you are serve as a "filter" that helps you consciously, or unconsciously, "choose" potentials out of the Quantum Field of Infinite Potential.

- If you want to start consciously choosing something better for your life, you have to start by changing your personal story.

- To do this, you need to start by understanding what your stories are telling you about key areas in your life. This gives you a starting place to rewrite your story.

- To create the energy that permanently transforms your story and protects you from default conditioned programming in your mind, body, and spirit, you have to work on all levels of the "manifesting equation."

- The biggest challenge you face when taking back control of your personal narrative and reclaiming your natural creative power, is to figure out exactly what stories you're telling. Which parts of your story do you need to change, in order to activate your potential and improve the quality of your life.

- If your story of who you are creates your experience of reality, then the most important question you need to be asking yourself is, who is the "you" creating your life? How do you create an energetically aligned way to untangle yourself from a story you are outgrowing?

The question of who you are is a challenging question and not always an easy one to answer. Historically, we have looked to stories, myths, and archetypes to help us identify with aspects of ourselves. Since the beginning of the human story, we've sat around fires, telling tales of heroes and tricksters who are simply archetypal aspects of characters that live within all of us to varying degrees. Ancient wisdom keepers created archetype-based personality systems such as astrology and numerology to determine who we are, how we are, and why we're here.

In modern times, we've turned to science to explain who we are. We've learned certain personality traits are inherited. We've discovered our DNA is more malleable than we thought. Changing the long-standing debate of nature vs. nurture. We learned the protein coats that regulate how our genes function (epigenes) contain ancestral "memories," which influence how we experience the world and, particularly, how we create wellness and well-being. We know our lived experiences, especially in our childhood, can influence our self-perception, our physiology, and even create ongoing trauma reactions that cause us to forget or hide who we are as a coping mechanism when we don't feel safe, valued, or accepted.

We learn the collective "formula" for being successful at an early age. Your parents, teachers, and society taught you vital lessons that shaped your desires, intentions, and even your definition of what it means to be successful and abundant. The cultural narrative, what you read in the news, saw on social media, and watched on TV showed you stories that inform the decisions you make about what to pursue, who to become, and what you need to do to create success in your life.

All of these elements, called "conditioning," contribute to the story of who you are. Trying to untangle your personal story from these elements can be tricky and sometimes scary. Defining and deconditioning your story often requires the courage to step out of your family and cultural narrative and take the risk of creating success on your own terms. For many of us, this means trusting we'll continue to be loved, valued, and accepted in the world, even if we don't follow all the rules the world has laid out for us.

It's no wonder most of us learn to play it safe! We put off defining our own story until we feel like we have nothing to lose and our foundation is strong and solid.

The good news is you no longer have to wait for random external circumstances, and the passage of time, to help you experience a foundation that is strong and solid. You can engineer these circumstances using scientifically supported modalities that work across all levels of manifesting.

When you work to shift your personal story on the quantum level, mental and emotional body level, subtle body level, and physical level, you create a dynamic, integrated matrix that helps you shift your personal story permanently. (And change your family "story" along the way so you can heal ancestral narratives in all directions of time)

If you're like most people, you've probably tried to improve your habits, change the way you think about things, and set goals to try to create optimal wellness. While all of these actions can result in a certain amount of growth and change, it's also pretty common for people to try to make big lifestyle, or mindset changes with little progress before defaulting back to old patterns and behaviors.

There are many reasons why we tend to go back to our default programming. The biggest reason is, that we are pretty efficient creatures. Once it establishes a pattern of behavior or thought, it tends to run to patterns pretty automatically via neural pathways and energy channels.

Neural pathways are a series of connected neurons that transmit signals from one part of the nervous system to another. These pathways allow for communication between different areas of the brain and between the brain and the rest of the body. Signals travel along the neurons in the form of electrical impulses, and these impulses are transmitted across synapses (gaps between neurons) through chemical messengers called neurotransmitters. Neural pathways enable us to think, feel, move, and perform various bodily functions in a relatively unconscious way.

Think about walking. Most of us aren't walking and thinking about which foot to put down as we take steps. We mindlessly move our bodies wherever we want to go. This is because, as we learn to walk as toddlers, our brain is building neural pathways that make walking an automatic event.

Anytime we want to establish a new habit, or set a new goal, we're basically "rewiring" the brain. Rewiring the brain without a healthy foundation for change requires tremendous willpower and the ability to stick with the new pattern long enough to make new neural pathways, even when all of your old default patterns and established pathways get triggered.

You can make the process of "rewiring" the brain much easier and "default-proof" when you consciously construct a multi-dimensional matrix to support the changes you're trying to make. An integrated approach to changing your story makes your new story resilient, rapidly shifts your point of creation, and avoids boom and bust cycles of motivation and burnout. The changes you make become enduring and permanent.

In addition, as you learned in the previous chapter, the brain is a manifestation on the physical level of a quantum potential influenced by the beliefs and memories held in your mental and emotional body and the energy channel established in your subtle body.

You are more than just a physical pattern. Your patterns are held on multiple levels of your being. To create truly effective and lasting change, you must address all of these levels.

I started my professional career as a Registered Nurse and a midwife. My career was immersed in the traditional healthcare system and deeply rooted in science. I struggled with the incongruity of a "health care" system that wasn't really helping people get permanently healthy. I have always been curious to explore how to best help people get out of pain.

In my quest to help people eliminate the root cause of their pain, I studied life coaching and became one of the very first coaches trained in the world. While learning to coach gave me powerful skills, it still didn't really give me the depth I was craving to help my clients experience permanent shifts. I spent a lot of time trying to "diagnose" the root cause of my client's challenges and not really finding the answers I needed to effectively help them.

At the same time, I also took a deep dive into holistic health traditions like The Emotional Freedom Techniques (EFT), flower essences, Healing Touch, healing sound frequencies, and other subtle body energy techniques. I knew I was sitting on a wealth of life-changing tools, but I still felt like my approach was "hit or miss," so I kept searching.

I then worked for and studied under Ra Uru Hu (the founder of Human Design) and learned the power of Human Design through my "healer" eyes. Human Design gave me a more targeted approach to all of the modalities I was trained in.

Certainly, Human Design helped me get my clients faster and better results. However, I knew following Human Design without integrating evidence-supported strategies wasn't giving me a complete system to accelerate my client's results and help them get out of pain permanently.

While pursuing my PhD in Integrative Medicine, I realized until we treat the WHOLE person at every level of "manifestation," we are limited in the quality of transformation that we can facilitate for our clients. Once I understood the power of Quantum Medicine, I knew I had to work with people in such a way that my own conditioning and my own biases didn't impact my client's capacity to tap into their ability to heal themselves.

My role was not to "heal" them but to help them tap into new potentials for well-being on a quantum level in their own way.

Just like a bowl full of eggs, butter, flour, cocoa powder, and sugar are meaningless until you put them all together to bake a melt-in-your-mouth chocolate mousse cake, so too are coaching and energy healing modalities when they're kept separate. When mixed together, you can achieve true alchemy and lasting change.

In 2015, I blended essential science-supported modalities into an integrated energy-aligning protocol called the Quantum Alignment System. This system allowed me to better support my clients in getting to the root cause of their pain, and helping them regain control over the story they tell themselves (and the world) about who they are and how they are.

When you follow Quantum Alignment System protocols, quantum leaps in progress can and do occur beyond any single modality I've ever tried before.

In the Quantum Alignment System, we blend together:

- Quantum Human Design
- Quantum Questioning
- Flower Essences
- Healing Sound Frequencies
- Intentional Storytelling (StoryLab)
- Coaching

While I'm a big fan of the modalities I integrated into the Quantum Alignment System, you don't have to use these specific modalities to create an integrated approach to creating lasting transformation. It is quite possible to use other modalities provided that you are using modalities that address changing the personal narrative on the quantum, mental and emotional body, subtle body, and physical layers.

QUANTUM HUMAN DESIGN: THE PHYSICAL LEVEL

Each system that makes up Quantum Human Design consists of archetypes. Archetypes are aspects of the common human experience. Archetypes are neutral roles or characteristics in our personal story. It isn't until we give these archetypes meaning that they become part of our experience of reality.

For example, let's look at the archetype of the "hermit." The definition of the archetype "hermit" is simply a person who lives in seclusion. A more modern definition might be a person who needs alone time to recharge, what we would call an introvert. The shadow of this archetype might be a person who retreats and hides away from life to the degree to which they fail to access healthy support or relationships.

Part of the story of this shadow expression of "hermit" might be this person has a hard time setting healthy boundaries and often finds themselves overwhelmed with the energy of others. Instead of asking for healthy space, they hide out instead and give up on having healthy relationships.

Another expression of "hermit" might be a young mother who lives far from her family, and is struggling with feeling "touched out" by her baby. She has no time for herself and is feeling overwhelmed. She needs some alone time to recharge but can't get any because she's isolated. Her underlying story might be one of feeling she's not worthy of paying money to have someone come help her with her baby a couple of afternoons a week or not being able to ask for additional help from her family because she feels guilty or ashamed she's having such a hard time.

These are both aspects of the archetype of "hermit" being lived out in modern life. What determines how we experience the archetypes that comprise the human story? Our own personal narrative and the meanings we give the parts of our own stories (archetypes) based on our conditioning influence how we interpret and, ultimately, choose our translation of reality.

The Quantum Human Design chart, calculated using your birthday, time, and location, gives you a "blueprint" for your unique human story. Even though you may experience all of the archetypes in the human story at some point in your life, this experience either comes from within yourself or through your personal and collective relationships. You are born to explore certain archetypes as part of your personal soul curriculum. So, going back to the "hermit" example, you have "hermit" archetypes in your Quantum Human Design chart; this means part of what you're designed to explore in your life is how to be a healthy "hermit," and set good boundaries. You need to take care of yourself if you're feeling overwhelmed and accept you need alone time to recharge your system.

Each one of the ancient and modern archetypal systems that are part of Quantum Human Design revolves around the idea that we have choices. Astrology simply lays out a curriculum of possibilities for your life based on the planetary weather and your innate nature. The Chinese I'Ching is all about guiding the "evolved" human to make conscious choices. The Hindu Chakra system is about awakening, and choosing to step off the wheel of karma. Judaic Kabbalah teaches how to make conscious choices to live in deeper alignment with the divinity within us. Even quantum physics shows us our expectation creates our experience of reality, and if we change our expectations, our experience of reality shifts in response.

According to Quantum Human Design, the placement of the planets at your birth encodes your body with the story of your potential. The moment of your birth gives you a "snapshot" of who you were born to be. It also tells you how you experience energy, especially in relationships, and where you may be vulnerable to certain shadow aspects of your story. Your chart reveals your strengths, your gifts, and your life purpose.

Your Quantum Human Design chart is an energy map that can be used to help you explore the sources of pain in your life. You are designed to live in alignment with the potential outlined in your chart. To live a life that is true to who you are born to be. If you stray from the chart or live "off the chart," and live a life misaligned with your authentic nature; you will experience pain. This pain can be physical, emotional, or spiritual. The more you live "off the chart," denying your true nature; the more pain you potentially experience.

Traditionally, we tend to treat pain as the problem. What Quantum Human Design gives you is a systematic, and elegant way to get to the root of pain so you can address not only the symptom but the cause. The chart can be a powerful way to explore exactly what parts of your personal story are out of sync with your potential.

In this respect, Quantum Human Design is a powerful story-telling tool that can help you intentionally rewrite your story as a way of bringing yourself back into alignment with the person you were born to be.

THE EMOTIONAL FREEDOM TECHNIQUES (EFT): MENTAL AND EMOTIONAL BODY LEVEL

The Emotional Freedom Techniques (EFT), often referred to as "tapping," is a form of psychological acupressure that involves tapping on specific meridian points on the body while focusing on a specific issue or emotion. EFT is a powerful tool that helps with mental and emotional shifts in perspective that help re-frame limiting beliefs and reduce stress and anxiety.

If you are new to EFT or have never tried it for yourself, you'll find instructions on how to do EFT on our Reader Resource Page.

SUBTLE BODY: FLOWER ESSENCES AND HEALING SOUND FREQUENCIES

Working with the Subtle Body is part of the healing equation that is often overlooked when integrating a new story. Making changes on the physical, mental, and emotional levels can be strengthened by adding subtle body modalities such as flower essences and healing sound frequencies.

Flower essences are a type of natural remedy derived from the vibrational energy of flowers. They are used in alternative and complementary medicine to address emotional/mental imbalances rather than physical ailments. In the Quantum Alignment System, we use flower essences custom-crafted to align with specific energy frequencies related to elements in the Quantum Human Design chart.

SOUND FREQUENCIES

Healing sound frequencies, also known as sound therapy or sound healing, work on the principle that sound vibrations can affect the body and mind in beneficial ways. Every part of the body has a natural frequency of vibration. When these frequencies are disrupted (due to stress, illness, or other factors), it can lead to disharmony and imbalance. Sound healing uses specific frequencies and rhythms to restore these natural vibrations and promote healing.

Certain sound frequencies can influence brainwave patterns. For instance, binaural beats, which involve playing slightly different frequencies in each ear, can help entrain brainwaves to desired states such as relaxation, focus, or meditation. This can enhance mental clarity, reduce stress, and improve sleep.

Sound therapy can also facilitate the release of stored emotions. Different tones and frequencies can evoke emotional responses, helping individuals to process and release pent-up feelings. The soothing nature of certain sounds can induce deep states of relaxation, reducing stress and anxiety. This can have a positive impact on overall health, as chronic stress is linked to numerous health issues. In the Quantum Alignment system, we have created recordings of specific sound frequencies that stabilize the energy field and "tune" the body to a frequency of vitality.

Both of these modalities are frequency-based protocols. In other words, they "tune" the body's energy field to an aligned frequency of energy so your vibration stays aligned with the positive physical, mental, and emotional changes you're making.

I like to think of these as "energy splints," holding the energy in place to support the changes you're making on all the other layers.

You'll find a sample *Sound Healing Frequency with instructions* on the Reader Resource page, along with instructions for how to order custom-blended Quantum Human Design Flower essences.

QUANTUM LEVEL: QUANTUM QUESTIONS

Interacting with the quantum field through questions, rather than answers, or affirmations aligns with the principles of quantum mechanics. Consciousness theories suggest our reality is influenced by observation and intention.

Here's why this approach might be beneficial:

- **Openness and Possibility:** Questions keep your mind open to possibilities, allowing for a broader range of outcomes. This aligns with the probabilistic nature of the quantum field, where multiple possibilities exist until observed.

- **Focus and Intention:** Questions help focus your attention and intention on specific aspects of your reality, which can influence the quantum field. Intention is thought to play a crucial role in collapsing the wave function to create a specific outcome.

- **Curiosity and Growth:** Asking questions fosters curiosity, continuous growth, encouraging exploration, and discovery. This aligns with the dynamic and evolving nature of the quantum field.

- **Non-Attachment:** Questions promote a state of non-attachment to specific outcomes, reducing resistance and allowing the quantum field to bring forth the best possible result. Affirmations and answers can sometimes create rigidity and limit possibilities.

By engaging with the quantum field through questions, you create a collaborative and creative process that harnesses the uncertainty, and potential of quantum mechanics to manifest desired outcomes.

By using these four levels of being, you cultivate radical shifts in patterns, and habits, that support optimal wellness and well-being. In the next section of the mini-ebook, you're going to explore the basics of the Quantum Alignment System so you can begin to explore how to align yourself with your natural state of vitality and begin to untangle yourself from patterns that may be burning you out and impacting your body.

CHAPTER 3

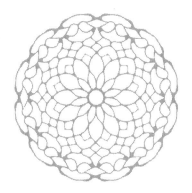

OVERVIEW OF QHD - TYPE/STRATEGY/AUTHORITY (AND THE QAS ALIGNMENT PROTOCOLS)

REVIEW:

- The stories you tell the world (and yourself) about who you are and how you are serve as a "filter" that helps you consciously, or unconsciously, "choose" potentials out of the Quantum Field of Infinite Potential.

- If you want to start consciously choosing something better for your life, you have to start first by changing your personal story.

- To do this, you need to start by understanding what stories you are telling right now about key areas in your life. This gives you a starting place to rewrite your story.

- To create the energy that helps transform your story permanently and protects you from default programming in your mind, body, and spirit, you have to work on all levels of the "manifesting equation."

- Once you prepare the energy to be receptive to a new personal story, the next step is to systematically explore the question, "Who are you, and who is the "you" who is creating your reality?

It takes a lot of energy to be someone you're not. Think of it like this. Imagine for a moment you are at a masquerade party holding up a Venetian mask. What are the odds you'll hold your mask up to your face all night? Even though the mask is lightweight, if you hold it up for any length of time, your arm is going to get stiff and tired. You'll eventually lower your arm and reveal your true face.

Anytime you say "yes" to something, you want to say "no" to it (and vice versa.) Anytime you lie about what you want and hide who you really are, it costs vital and precious energy. Eventually, this puts you at risk for burnout. If you've internalized from your life experiences it's somehow not okay or safe to be who you are or how you are, you will eventually spend your precious energy protecting your identity. Over time, your body may begin to pay the cost of inauthentic living.

The most important thing you can do right now to support the creation of a vital, vibrant, and healthy life is to begin a systematic exploration of the meanings you hold about who you are, why you're here, and what you're capable of.

The most significant thing you can do to begin to activate your innate creative power and create optimal wellness is to untangle yourself from old collective and personal beliefs about lack or limitation. Quantum Human Design is a powerful system that can help you explore your personal narrative in a systematic way so you discover who you are, how you operate, and how to begin telling yourself(and the world) a more aligned, authentic story.

In this chapter, you're going to learn the basics about Quantum Human Design in the context of your personal story. You're going to explore the archetypes in your chart as a way of systematically analyzing your story. This analysis will help you interpret the messages your body may be giving you and as a way to support you in creating optimal wellness and well-being.

The Quantum Human Design chart reveals layers in your personal story. Each layer gives you more refined and in-depth nuances. Each of these layers is composed of archetypes. As you explore the layers in more depth, you will be able to look at the spectrum of how you are experiencing this archetype in your life.

Are you living the "high" expression or the "low" expression? What needs to change in your story and in your life to consciously choose the highest expression of all the parts of your story? The quality of well-being in your body is often associated with the quality of how you are expressing the archetypal parts of your story.

Quantum Human Design is a powerful storytelling tool that gives you a system of "layers," helping you understand who is the YOU who is creating your experience of reality. The layers of the chart include the Nine Resiliency Keys, your Type, your Profile, your Centers, the Circuits and the Gates.

You'll be using the layers in your chart to help you systematically explore your personal story and, ultimately, rewrite your story to optimize your capacity to create optimal wellness and well-being.

Every story has a main character who is challenged and eventually grows and evolves. The main character usually starts the story living out the conditioned aspect of their story. As they experience the "adventure" of their story, they begin the process of deconditioning their identity becoming a more authentic and fulfilled version of themselves- the "hero" of the story.

As we explore the main character layer in your Quantum Human Design chart, I want you to think about this layer in the context of the story of your life. Many of my clients start out their journey with a deeply conditioned story.

They are pushing and trying to fit into their family and cultural narrative. They create according to the rules and formulas they've been taught to create success. Often, they encounter Quantum Human Design when they are exhausted and burned out. Unable to push against their authentic selves anymore.

TYPE: THE MAIN CHARACTER IN YOUR STORY

There are five main character Types in Quantum Human Design. Each Type has a unique role to play in the world, a specific way of making decisions, and distinct challenges they must overcome to fulfill the full potential of their role. Each Type is also vulnerable to burnout when they don't follow their unique energy flow.

As you explore your Type, you're going to learn about how your Type usually internalizes conditioning. You'll learn exactly what needs to happen in order to heal your connection to your body and the messages it is giving you. You'll discover what bringing your "main character" back to Baseline looks and feels like. You'll also learn about the highest expression, the Quantum Purpose, of your Type.

THE MANIFESTOR → INITIATOR

You are an Initiator. By following your inner timing and impulses, you create opportunities for yourself and others. When you live true to yourself, you create an energy field that inspires others to live more authentically. This isn't anything you say; it's the energy your authenticity creates. You are here to fully embody your direct, often non-verbal, connection to your authentic creativity. When you do, you have the potential to be a powerhouse of impact and influence.

You are the only Type designed to initiate action, but only when the timing feels right. Your inner sense of timing and your physical connection to how your body feels when things are "right" is essential for you.

It is vital to develop the sense of knowing your right timing; it's unnecessary for you to wait for outside confirmation before taking action. Your creative impulses come from inside of yourself. In spite of this ability to initiate, many Initiators have their personal way of interacting with the flow of life. They wait for signs in their outer world to tell them the timing is right to act.

Your biggest challenge is to remember what it feels like for you when it feels "right" to act.

Initiators are powerful, creative beings. As an Initiator, you have an internal, non-verbal creative flow that moves quickly when the timing is correct. This creative flow is so fast you often don't have time to put words to it. This lack of words often means when you intuitively sense the timing is right for you to act--you can just get up and get to it.

Your energy field carries with it the power to initiate others into action. When people are in your energy, they are often unconsciously poised, meaning they are ready to leap and get things going. Because of this frequency of energy, people pay attention to you and are always waiting to see what you do next.

As soon as you take action, other people usually notice, and will often interrupt your creative flow. They ask you if you need help or want to know what you're doing. They're not interrupting you because they are trying to stop you. Rather, it's just they sense something is about to happen, and they feel the need to be a part of it (or to be ready for what's next).

This interruption and these questions can be very difficult for your Initiator energy. Remember, you have an internal, non-verbal creative flow that you are following. It's an inner, gut-level sense of flow. When you have to stop that flow to find the words to explain to someone what you're doing, or you don't need help, it's often hard to find your creative flow in the same way again.

When you don't understand how your energy works, it's so easy to react with anger towards others. Other people can also become angry with you because they feel you aren't involving them (or sometimes being considerate of them) when they don't know what you're doing.

As a way of dealing with your energy, others may want to help you. This is their need to feel useful, but it's not your obligation to fulfill this need. You may find if you are trying to keep others happy to avoid the anger or other people's attempt to control you, you may feel disconnected from your creative power.

You may have developed elaborate strategies to secretly do what you want to do without the interference of others. Not being upfront and honest, as hard as it can be, uses up a lot of energy and can make you feel exhausted whenever you feel like you have to deal with people.

You could be done with what you're doing, in the time it can take you to find the right words and try to explain to someone what you're doing. But you'll lose your speed if you don't stop and inform the people who will be impacted by your creative flow what you're going to do next.

The trick for you, if you're an Initiator, is learning to honor your inner creative flow, and letting the people who will be impacted by your actions know what you're doing. Informing is NOT asking permission. You're not here to ask people for permission.

Learning to honor your creative flow, informing others, and not letting other people's discomfort with your choices is often the greatest place of learning for Initiators.

CONDITIONED EXPRESSION:

As an Initiator, you can become depleted, angry, and burned out when disconnected from your internal flow. When disconnected, your innate connection to your authentic creative impulses, and your need for inner alignment before taking action are also depleted. This disconnect from your authentic self creates a conditioned experience of using your tremendous initiating capacity to try to push or force life circumstances.

This pushing against your own inner flow is exhausting and creates a chronic state of creative disruption in your life. Leaving you feeling like you aren't fulfilling your full potential. In order to avoid other people's judgment or input on your creative process, you may have learned to quietly do your own thing on the side, or to give up your own desires altogether.

Working regular "9-5 hours" or more is very difficult and unnatural for the Initiator. As an Initiator, you need to be very conscious about structuring your business or your work around your energy because you don't have sustainable energy for work. Your energy tends to be cyclical with a deep need for rest cycles in between bursts of creative energy.

Initiators don't usually make good team players and tend to want to do everything themselves. Delegating can be hard for the Initiator / Manifestor because it feels "faster" to do it yourself. Finding the words for your creative flow slows you down and feels unnatural.

Initiators have a unique energy that makes it easier for them to get things started. Sometimes, when you're an Initiator, it's easy to lose your patience with other people who simply are not hard-wired the way you are.

It can also be difficult, once you get something started, to follow through with the energy to bring it to completion, or to manage your creation on a day-to-day level. Remember, you're an initiator, not necessarily a "do-er."

Initiators do NOT have sustainable life and workforce energy. This lack of access is why most Initiators are not particularly good at seeing a project or fulfilling an idea, to its end. You're not here to do the deep detail work. You're here to start the expression of an idea and then hand off the details to others to complete. As an Initiator, you are not designed to finish the sustained implementation of ideas and projects.

The follow-through and maintenance tasks are not in your Type. Yours is a creative and initiating energy. You originate opportunities and move on to create the next.

Initiators give the rest of us reasons to respond—you are like the cue ball on a pool table, bumping into the other balls and causing them to move.

STRATEGY: TO INFORM

Each Type has a unique Strategy, a way of being in the world that begins the process of helping you move from the Conditioned Expression of your energy, to the Baseline of your energy. For you as a Manifestor, the most important thing to do for you to heal is to reconnect to your body. Reconnect how it feels, inside your body, when your creative flow and right timing are aligned.

This takes practice.

It's also essential you remember you're here to follow your flow. Because you most likely have old stories around needing to tailor your creative flow to please others, you have to remember how to follow your flow and stop caring about pleasing others. Even though you may have been trained that this is deeply selfish, it's actually beneficial for the people you love for you to be authentic and in your creative flow. You are not the problem. The problem might be you need to teach people about who you are, how you are, AND you need to surround yourself with people who support and understand your creative power. The right people for you will simply move out of your way and celebrate you following your creative flow.

If you are an Initiator, it's correct for you to start things, not necessarily implement the details or finish the projects. You must learn to delegate and/or move on when it feels correct to do so.

If you're feeling stuck or "shut down," start initiating more in your life. It's okay to start with small tasks and projects to rebuild that "initiating muscle." After all, it may have been suppressed for most (if not all) of your life. You'll feel MUCH better when you are behaving the way you are designed to behave. And you'll have more energy.

As an Initiator, your energy field impacts others deeply. Because of this, people notice you and can often sense when you are about to spring into action. This can cause people to either ask if they can help you or question what you're doing.

Your internal, non-verbal creative flow can cause you to struggle with translating what you're about to do into words. Stopping to explain what you're doing, or that you don't need help, can cause you to lose your connection to your internal non-verbal creative flow. As unnatural as it can seem, when you inform those people that your actions will have an impact on what you're about to do, it can actually prepare the way for you to follow your creative flow with minimal disruption and drama.

It takes courage to do this; it will take time for it to become a habit but will be worth it. Your relationships and even your health and wellness will improve because of it. It will also minimize the amount of anger and resistance that you experience from others.

Informing isn't asking permission. You don't need permission. Don't be afraid of others saying no, or trying to stop you. You can still do as intended, but it'll be wise to take others' views into consideration if you can-there's nothing wrong with a second opinion!

Informing simply allows people to move out of your way and support you so you can do what you feel inspired to do. Your natural alignment with your inner creative flow ultimately benefits everyone around you.

Recognize the impact you have on people around you. You have a very strong and powerful aura. Others will usually feel your presence when you enter a room. Some Initiators / Manifestors are surprised to learn this about themselves, but the people around them know it to be true.

Trust what 'feels' right to you (not just what your brain-based analysis tells you). Manage your energy and take breaks when needed. Don't try to keep up with the sustainable energy of the 70% of the population who do have consistent Sacral energy.

It's MUCH easier to avoid burnout than to recover from it!

Initiators can initiate action and opportunity without waiting. You are an energy being that possesses tremendous initiating power, but you have to use your power carefully or risk angering others.

Your purpose in life is to create action for a reaction. If an Initiator decides to start a business all they have to do is decide on the right timing, and then just do it.

Although most of us think we would love to be Initiators, being an Initiator can have its own challenges. Many Initiators have struggled to learn to use their power appropriately and may be conditioned to hide their power (or suppress it entirely.)

You must learn how to channel your energy properly, or you will face tremendous resistance in life. Properly channeled Initiator energy initiates the people around you to tap into their own creativity and authentic self-expression.

Without informing, you will get resistance every step of the way. That's why many Initiators (starting in their childhood) resign after being punished repeatedly by parents, teachers, and others who don't understand the power of the Initiator.

When Initiators give up their manifesting powers, they surrender to going through life just getting by. If you do this, you may feel ignored or like you've been run over by a truck. The last thing you would want to do is to inform others. Everybody else is in your way all the time, so the idea of making it easier for others by informing is unacceptable. Yet, it's the only way out of the cycle of control and resistance. (While still living with parents, Initiators' (Manifestors') strategy is actually different - they need to ask for permission.)

Over time, as you reconnect with your inner power and the way your creative flow feels inside of you, your outer life will change. The people in your life will begin to see you differently and will understand they simply need to move out of the way when you're in your creative flow. Your energy will be exciting and dynamic. People will naturally be ready for you. As you integrate your power, your Quantum Purpose of lifting the energy in the room and showing others what authentic creativity and power looks like will deepen. You will become a powerful influence and have a deep impact on others.

EMOTIONAL THEME: ANGER

You can experience anger in your life, either from within or from others, when your creative flow gets disrupted. Your anger really isn't what we typically think of as anger as much as it's the result of your creative energy being interrupted. Your energy becomes dissipated because it didn't get to fulfill its purpose.

If you get interrupted while you're in the process of creating, that energy has to go somewhere, and you may often experience it as a feeling of anger. Think of it like this: your creative flow is as powerful as a volcano. If that movement of energy gets disrupted, or blocked, it explodes. Your "anger" is simply an expression of creative disruption.

Other people can also be angry with you when you fail to inform them, and they don't understand what you're doing. It's normal for you to experience anger periodically. If you are experiencing chronic anger in your life, it's important to explore if your natural creative flow is being supported and honored by yourself and those around you.

Initiators often struggle with knowing when enough is enough. If you're an Initiator, it's important to gauge what you're doing and make sure you're not frying everyone else's energy causing them to burn out. If you are, that doesn't mean you should stop what you're doing, but be aware sometimes this may trigger anger in others.

On an energetic level, you have quite the impression on others, but your aura doesn't communicate as much as the auras of other types. Because of this, others are not sure how to accept you, which is why communication is so important.

Inform those in your circle of influence. This is how to release the tension others may feel about you. By bringing them into the conversation, they may help you and put their energy into whatever it is that you have initiated. At that point, you will find what you've been seeking, the completion of your creative inspiration.

WORK

The design of Initiators can affect relationships in work and life choices.

Initiators CAN and DO have jobs, or businesses, and raise families. However, you may burn out around age 50 (or before) if you continue attempting to accomplish too much, especially if pushing yourself to keep up with the 70% of the population who have consistent Sacral energy.

Initiators don't "need" people the way other Types need people, which affects how you operate within relationships. The biggest challenge (and a key piece of your Strategy for success in life) is INFORMING those who are affected by your actions before acting and making sure the people in your life are healthy and don't tie their self-worth to your actions.

More so than other Types, Initiators don't like being told what to do. If you feel obligated to ask permission to do something or feel manipulated in any way, you may become overly defiant and angry towards or feel repressed by others, turning those feelings inward and creating anxiety, depression, or even illness. You need people in your life who accept you and honor your creative power.

HEALTH

For Initiators to stay healthy, they need to be powerful. If you have not been using your power, or if you've shut yourself off from your Initiator energy, your energy doesn't go away. It ricochets inside your body either burning you out or sometimes creating depression and anxiety.

If you have a lifetime of using your power without informing others, if you have fought and struggled to keep people out of your way so you can do what you feel like you need to do, then you may also experience burnout.

Many Initiators burn out around the age of 50 if they haven't been using their energy properly. Burnout can come from not knowing when enough is enough, pushing without the balance of rest, trying to work in ways that are not in alignment with your energy, and denying your own power.

If you're burned out, the number one priority in your life is healing the burnout. Often, that means stopping everything in your life and catching up on the rest you need to restore and recharge your energy.

Getting good, healthy sleep is of particular importance for Initiators, and to do so, you need to lie down before you feel tired. You can read or watch a movie for a while before you fall asleep, but lying in a horizontal position. Being flat in a horizontal position allows you to release the energy you've taken in during the day and helps your body discharge excess energy.

If possible, sleep alone, not in range of other people's aura. If you can do this, you will feel the difference in the morning. If you share a house or live in an apartment, remember there may be a neighbor above or behind the wall where you are sleeping. If you're closer than your two arm-lengths, you are still in each other's aura.

You'll sleep better if you can reposition your bed to be as far away from the energy of others as possible.

QUANTUM EXPRESSION:

An awakened Initiator is deeply connected to Divine Inspiration and the flow of Spirit; as the result of a deep connection to the value of the unique role that only the Initiator can play. A masterful Initiator is aware of their power, informs those who their actions will impact, and moves forward when the timing is right. They own their power, and never allow

37

the judgment of others to impede their creative flow. They are honoring and aware of the initiating force they bring to the world. They serve the Creative Muse and are transformational agents of change.

The initiation you bring isn't really about what you "do." Ultimately, it is through your modeling for the world what alignment and authentic living looks like that people feel inspired to do the same for themselves- in their unique way.

Relentlessly expressing your authentic self, inspires and initiates the people around you.

LESSON/CHALLENGE:

The challenge of the Initiator is to learn to use their creative essence sustainably. To be sustainable and to truly serve their purpose of initiating others, the Initiator must heal their relationship with their personal power, reclaim their power, cultivate an internal alignment with their truth, their creative flow, and learn to be at peace with the idea that they are uniquely connected to a creative force in a way that not many others share.

Once an Initiator can integrate the value of their power and their role in the world, they can also heal their feelings of being alone and embrace their unique role in waking the world.

AFFIRMATION:

I am a powerful creative force. I trust my inner sense of timing to act on my creative intentions. I follow my creative flow and inform those who may be impacted by my actions so that they can support me and clear the path for me to do what I need to do. I recognize my value and know that when I follow my creative flow. I am not only bringing something new into the world, I am initiating others into new possibilities. I value the unique role only I can play. I honor my power and commit to nurturing my energy, so I can act with great power when the timing is correct. I am a transformational force, and my actions change the world.

Some famous Initiators include Al Gore, George W. Bush, Jack Nicholson, Susan Sarandon, Richard Burton, and Vladamir Putin.

THE GENERATOR → ALCHEMIST

You are an Alchemist. You are designed to learn and achieve mastery over the physical plane. Your life is a series of adventures that help you learn through practice, exploration, and experience.

By learning to trust your gut and follow what feels right and aligned, you are designed to delight in your learning. You need work, and opportunities that feel good and important to you. When you are engaged with work that is fulfilling, you tap into a quality of life-force energy that is enduring and gives you energy and momentum.

Alchemists play the part of patient seekers who become fully activated in their life purpose when they learn to respond to what the world brings them instead of trying to "figure out" with their minds what they should be doing. The Alchemists have the potential to be Masters of what they respond to do and to create.

Alchemists know they hold this energy. As you're an Alchemist Type, you often feel frustrated because you can sense deep inside of yourself that you're here to do something that fulfills your full potential. If your life feels meaningless and you feel unfulfilled, it is an internal sign that you're not living true to your authentic nature.

As an Alchemist, you're trained by the world to use your thinking and the power of your mind to set your path to mastery. The truth for Alchemists is that the path is revealed to you by the world outside of yourself. It takes faith and the understanding of how to connect with that path correctly to align yourself with your destiny and the ultimate fulfillment of your potential.

You have to wait for something outside of yourself to confirm that:

• Your idea IS actually the right idea for you.

• The timing is now right to take action on your idea.

• Your gut senses that what is showing up in your life feels good, right and aligned.

Over time, as you heal, reconnect, and learn to trust your gut, you don't necessarily have to wait for confirmation from your outer world. You will learn to know the difference between the voices in your head that are rooted in hidden agendas like proving your worth to the world, versus your pure connection to inspiration. Your job, as you reconnect with your body, is to reconnect with pure inspiration, and to tune into the wisdom of your body to let you know how and when to follow what inspires you. When you reawaken, you become the Alchemist; turning inspiration into form and joyfully doing the "work" to create on the physical plane.

CONDITIONED EXPRESSION:

The Alchemist in the conditioned expression runs like an endless, indiscriminate source of energy that is "all revved up" with nowhere to go. Generating energy without direction or efficiency.

Much like a generator that you might run when the power is out, you need a source of energy to keep going. When you feel disconnected from the work of the world that is meaningful and relevant to your life, you can eventually run "out of gas." It's common for you to quit repeatedly and feel frustrated when you don't know how to dial into your "gut feelings" and follow what feels relevant and right to you.

Most Alchemists have been taught to bypass their own inner wisdom and to adopt a "just do it" attitude about the things they think they "should" be doing. Alchemists may find it difficult to refrain from "just doing it" because it requires ignoring old ideas about hard work, success, and money. It can feel scary, or even irresponsible to follow your gut (your inner wisdom) and forego the programming of your mind.

As an Alchemist, you are an energy being. You have the energy to work; even at jobs you hate. Sadly, many Alchemists do this for their entire lives.

When an Alchemist is simply working, but not working at a job they responded to, they fail to tap into the full expression of their potential and the vital life-force energy that turns on when they respond to doing the work that feels right. This isn't just about a job for money. This is about your life's work, which can also include doing service, taking care of a family, or whatever other inspirations turn you "on."

When an Alchemist hastily responds and doesn't realize that mastery takes time, and repetition as part of natural cycles of growth, then frustration and burnout eventually ensue. It's not until you learn to be patient and withhold pursuing what you "think" you should be doing, and let your life path unfold in front of you that the energy appears. In essence, it's like waiting for a "sign" or a signal that the timing must be right before acting.

When an Alchemist allows themselves to wait, they create a magical force that attracts everyone around them. When you, as an Alchemist, wait, you create an energy that will continue to grow until your true purpose appears. Your outer world begins to point the way to your next cycle of growth, or your next learning adventure.

Every Alchemist has a fear that if you do nothing and wait--nothing will happen. But every Alchemist who has the courage to wait soon sees that this fear is unfounded. You are in a constant dance with the Universe. Your life and the world around you are part of a divine feedback loop. When you follow the things that feel good and "right," you'll learn what is next for you, and you'll discover what you need to do next.

When an Alchemist waits and steps into their full purpose and potential, you wake up to the vitality and joy that you've been waiting for your whole life.

STRATEGY: WAIT TO RESPOND

Each Type has a unique Strategy, a way of being in the world that begins the process of helping you move from the Conditioned Expression of your energy to the Baseline of your energy. As an Alchemist, you have an inner compass called your Sacral (your "gut feeling") The Sacral lets you know when an opportunity feels right.

You're designed to follow what feels good. Sometimes, Alchemists have to re-learn how to trust that inner feeling. Your logical mind, and your cultural conditioning, may have trained you to ignore this vital inner compass and default to using your mind to resolve your challenges or "figure out" your next right step.

Alchemists can find themselves being confined to work they hate, feeling the drudgery of routine without joy, lost in unproductive labor, feeling there is something missing, knowing they may have made a mistake, and not knowing how to get out. Ultimately, if you are doing this you will burn out, or live life at a level of compromise, which will create more and more frustration, or simply have a life of quiet despair.

Your Sacral works best when you wait to see what shows up in your life and then allow yourself to follow the things that feel good. It can feel hard to wait to respond because you've been trained to go out and "make it happen." If you slow down, and wait, and see what shows up in your life, and then "feel" your way into it, you will slowly recover your connection to the inner wisdom of your body.

The Alchemist Strategy is to wait to respond. This is a simple, although often confusing aspect for the Alchemist. "Wait to respond" simply means that even if you have an incredibly inspiring insight, thought, or idea, you need to wait for confirmation in your outer world before you take action until you eventually learn to "feel" which of these ideas is actually right for you.

Confirmation in your outside world can be someone saying something to you, a "sign" from the Universe, or some kind of physical initiation that comes from outside of your mind. Once you get the "sign" or something to which you know you should respond, you can then act on the inspirations that feel good and right. Learning to follow the signs is kind of like training wheels for remembering how your body feels when something feels right (or wrong.) The more you wait and allow yourself to sense what feels right, the more you reconnect to the wisdom of your body so you can begin to trust yourself again.

As an Alchemist, in order to find your path, you have to learn how to use your energy correctly. Alchemist Types are the only Types who have a defined Sacral Motor. The Sacral Motor is the source of a direction-giving, nonverbal, gut-level vibration that tells you what feels right and what doesn't.

You may experience the Sacral response as a "gut feeling," and you can connect with it even more deeply when you express that "gut feeling" with a non-verbal sound. The "Sacral Sound" sounds like "uh-huh" for a "yes" and "un-uhn" for a "no."

Most Alchemists naturally make these sounds, but during childhood are often taught that they are rude, and to "use our words instead." When you watch Alchemist children, you'll notice that they are grunting, humming, sound-based beings. When you lose touch with the power of these sounds, you lose touch with your special inner compass that is designed to signal you to show you which direction is yours to follow.

This Sacral Sound is the sound of your inner intuition; the vibrational alignment with your correct direction in life. It is that direction that will take you to the next step in the unfolding of your mastery. The

Sacral is the truth. The Sacral cannot lie.

The Sacral Center is a source of sustainable energy. All of the motors in the Human Design System, except for the Sacral, have wave-like, inconsistent qualities, but the Sacral keeps going and going. It is sustainable energy for work, and life-force. It's about providing: resources, education, children, taking care of the family, the tribe, and the community.

Alchemists have two primary focuses in life: work and family. As an Alchemist, you will feel most fulfilled when you are pursuing one, or both, of these focuses.

For Alchemists, life is about RESPONSE. Instead of chasing after an inauthentic life, Alchemists must be patient and allow an authentic life to appear. The goal of an Alchemist is to discover, pursue, and dedicate their life to what they love.

EMOTIONAL THEME: FRUSTRATION

We're taught that learning and mastery is a linear process. The more effort you put into it, the more you learn, and the better you get. This just isn't true for you, my dear Alchemist!

The Emotional Theme for the Alchemist is frustration. You may experience two different kinds of frustration. The first source of frustration for the Alchemist comes from feeling "stuck" or trapped in a life that feels meaningless, and misaligned. You may feel and sense you have a greater potential than what you're tapping into, and this can feel deeply frustrating. If you are an Alchemist experiencing chronic frustration, you may eventually find yourself burned out and living a mediocre life. This will eventually take a toll on your physical well-being.

There is a second source of natural frustration for an Alchemist. You have a "stair-step" style learning curve. When you learn something new, you have an initial surge in mastery. You get good at whatever you're learning in record time. Once you reach a certain level, it's normal for you to sit on a plateau; where no matter how hard you try, you feel stuck, and like you're not making any progress.

Because you have a "stair-step" learning curve, it is normal that once you respond to a new opportunity there will be a surge in mastery. It feels good to be doing or learning something new, and you can learn quickly. Eventually, all Alchemists hit a plateau. It can feel like you're "stuck" and that nothing is happening.

43

This is when you feel frustrated, and you quit. Frustration may have caused you to become a serial quitter. Leaping from thing to thing, trying to find satisfying, meaning, and fulfilling work to do in the world.

Plateaus are normal for you! The challenge is learning how to work with the frustration that comes with plateaus. Frustration is often a symptom of energy building and momentum gathering for the next surge in mastery. You may have had the experience of waking up and suddenly finding your skills improved even though it seems like you didn't do anything to improve them.

Being on plateaus is a phase of learning, energy integration, and growth. The plateau can be dangerous for the Alchemist who doesn't understand their unique energy. The tendency for many Alchemists is to quit when they are on the plateau; failing to recognize that the plateau is simply a normal part of your process.

When the Alchemist understands that the plateau is the moment to wait for the next opportunity to respond to, they find their mastery. Frustration can simply be a sign that it is time to wait.

The "uh-huh" and the "un-unh" sounds turn on the Sacral Motor. That's your truth. This sound-based "gut feeling" is unique to the Alchemists. The gut is the source of the truth, and helps you bypass your conditioned thoughts and reconnect with the wisdom of the body. You must ask questions of yourself and monitor your gut response with the "uh-huh" and "un-unh." When you aren't responding and trying to force things into creation, you will most likely experience frustration.

The Sacral is a tremendous generator that provides energy. Sacral energy is enough to do all things when you follow that gut pulse. Alchemists who don't respond to the energy end up deeply frustrated. It's imperative to remain patient, and recognize the presence of the energy when it appears. The power of the defined Sacral Center will lead the way to one's true life purpose. Trust your inner response (Sacral). The Sacral Center provides Alchemists with a virtually inexhaustible source of energy.

If you quit instead of waiting, you may miss the next aligned opportunity for your growth and mastery. Instead, you spend a lifetime of starting and quitting and starting and quitting, never getting to be masterful at what you are really created to do.

SATISFACTION is a keyword for Alchemists. It's all about tapping into your sacral energies that open the door to the satisfaction of work and family. Your Sacral response will take you to where you can experience the greatest satisfaction, vitality, and joy.

HEALTH

Your brain will often work hard to figure out the right answers, but that is NOT where YOU want to be making your decisions. Decisions are what your Sacral responses are for. Alchemists who have not tuned into their Sacral are vulnerable to burnout. Not being true to your energy and trying to do something that doesn't satisfy you can (and will) make you exhausted.

Here are some ways that Alchemists can lose energy or burnout:

- Not loving work or environment.
- Sedentary lifestyle.
- Not following their Sacral guidance.
- Over-exerting themselves and not recharging their energy.
- Feeling frustrated and impatient when results aren't quickly realized.

As an Alchemist you have your own inner guidance system (Sacral) that can tell you what you need to do for health and wellness. It has to feel right and aligned with your Sacral to commit to a health and wellness routine.

As energy beings, Alchemists need a lot of movement and exercise to burn off excess energy. Alchemists who are struggling with insomnia or poor-quality sleep can benefit from more physical activity.

QUANTUM EXPRESSION:

The goal of the Alchemist is to achieve mastery. You cannot achieve mastery if you're leaping into things that don't feel right. You cannot be the master you are designed to be if you are afraid to trust the unfolding of your life, and the abundance of the Universe.

It is the Alchemist's job to take inspiration, and give it form through creative work. The Alchemists build the manifested form of Cosmic Order, and when you follow your Sacral impulses, you are led to your right place and true destiny in the world.

The masterful Alchemist understands their life is an arena within which they explore their mastery. Through responding, enduring, sustaining, practice, repetition, and correction, the Alchemist learns who they are and how they best respond to life. They use their life to fully embody the story of who they are.

The Alchemist understands that there is no "figuring out" their next right step. They cultivate a deep and aligned relationship with their purpose and path, and trust that the next level of mastery will be revealed to them when they are ready.

It is through allowing, and responding, the Alchemist learns to fulfill their life's purpose. Their deep connection to their Sacral will enable them to either stay with an experience, and continue to grow in mastery, or to accept that they have gleaned the necessary lessons and it is time to wait for the next opportunity for growth. The spiritual challenge of the Alchemist is to trust the unfolding of the Divine Order and your place within it.

LESSON/CHALLENGE:

To learn to wait for the next right step. To master the ability to sit with and be with your frustration; recognizing that frustration signals your momentum for change is growing. To learn to trust your inner Sacral response and how your body responds to what feels right, or wrong. Allow the trajectory of your mastery to unfold with ease and grace.

AFFIRMATION:

My life gives me an arena within which to explore myself and who I am. I let my inner alignment with my truth, and what feels right, guide me, and reveal the next right step. I strengthen my self-trust, and courage, so I can confidently follow my path. I use the power of my mind to inspire me and allow for the gentle unfolding of my life path. I trust in the cycles of growth in my life, knowing that my destiny is to be the fulfillment of who I am. I listen to the signal that frustration gives me, knowing that my frustration informs me that change is coming.

Famous Alchemists: Albert Einstein, Dalai Lama, Elvis Presley, Bill Clinton, Meryl Streep, John Lennon, Madonna, Vladimir Lenin, Carl Jung, Timothy Leary, Oprah Winfrey, Meg Ryan, Margaret Thatcher, Deepak Chopra, Jay Z, and Kim Kardashian.

THE MANIFESTING GENERATOR →TIME BENDER

You are a Time Bender. Your role in life is to find the fastest, most effective way to do things. You're a hybrid Type, part Initiator, part Alchemist. Like the Alchemist, you are designed to learn, and achieve mastery, over the physical plane. Like the Initiator, you have an internal, non-verbal creative flow that sets you in motion when you sense that the timing is right. (Be sure to read the section about the Initiator and the Alchemist in addition to this section.)

Your life is a series of learning adventures. Through practice, exploration, experience, and learning to trust your gut to follow what feels right and aligned; you are designed to delight in your learning. You're also designed to find the quickest path to mastery. You need work that feels good and is important to you. When you're engaged with work that is fulfilling, you tap into a quality of life-force energy that is enduring and gives you energy and momentum.

You can leap into it quickly when you find the work that delights and feels right to you. You have an internal, non-verbal creative flow that often makes it hard for you to explain what you're doing to others.

You have a tendency to do more than one thing at a time, and this is correct for you. You've probably been told to pick one thing to focus on all of your life, but that is just not true for you. You need to be engaged with multiple opportunities to occupy the massive amount of energy you carry.

However, not everything you try will be successful by society's definition. Some of the things you try, will teach you what you need to learn, even if they don't yield the results you had hoped.

You may also have a tendency to skip steps. That's okay! This is part of you finding the fastest path. Sometimes you have to go back and fix steps you skipped, but that doesn't mean you screwed up.

Time Benders have a deep inner awareness to know what's right for them as they wait for a "sign," or a signal, that the timing is right to act. A strong intuition turned on by gut-level pulses will place Time Benders in the right place, doing the right work, and having the right impact.

Even though you may feel like you know what you're doing and that you're wildly capable of doing all the things you're engaged with, others may often find your speed and your multitasking problematic. Your challenge is to relearn to trust yourself and to reconnect with the wisdom of your "gut feelings" and hunches.

The Time Bender explodes with frustration and anger when they can feel their energy could be used to fulfill their purpose, but they don't remember how to engage with direction and purpose. When the Time Bender is disconnected from their true purpose, they are "all revved" with nowhere to go. You have a built-in source of "backup" energy. When you push against your inner flow, and the outer unfolding of your trajectory, it can leave you feeling profoundly unfulfilled.

Time Benders can feel chronically "stuck." They feel frustrated and angry if they shut down their experiments to find the fastest, most efficient way. They can also feel this way if they limit what they do and try to slow themselves down, because others have told them that the way they do things is "wrong," sloppy, or careless.

Patience is extremely important for the Time Bender. The process of re-learning how to read the cues your body is sending can feel deeply frustrating and epically slow. When it is time for you to leap into action, your energy carries a lot of impact and can confuse, or overwhelm, those around you. Your creative flow is non-verbal and internal. If the people around you try to help you, or ask you questions, it can cause you to lose your connection to flow and you may react with anger and frustration. Because of this, especially in the beginning, when you're re-learning how to connect with your body's wisdom, you need to pay attention to who is in your "impact field" of action, and inform those around you about what you're about to do. This is NOT asking permission or even asking for help. Informing is simply about preparing the people around you for the impact of your actions and energy.

If you experience chronic frustration and anger, it may be that you're either pushing towards creating things out of alignment with what feels right, or you may have surrounded yourself with people who don't know how to support your creative process.

As a Time Bender, it may seem that you continually change your mind. For you, the need to internally check responses as you respond to situations confirms if what you've started is "still good for you." In essence, it's like waiting for a "sign," or a signal, that the timing is right before taking action.

Sometimes, Time Benders get out of balance. You love your work so much you forget to come up for air. Time Benders move very fast and often have a hard time being team players, preferring to work on their own. Delegating and letting go can be challenging. You often need help "triaging" your time and energy to make sure you're not doing everything just because you can.

Time Benders and Alchemists must recognize that finding the right work is the most important thing in life. Burnout occurs if you, as a Time Bender, aren't working on something you love. If satisfaction isn't found for the Time Bender, frustration and unhappiness take hold. In contrast, when you realize your true work, the Sacral Center provides you with a virtually inexhaustible source of energy.

Time Benders determine the fastest way to complete tasks, often skipping steps in the process while getting things "done." If you find those skipped steps to be important, you will eventually circle back to complete them. You skip steps because you're experimenting with finding the fastest way. You literally NEED to skip steps as part of your experiment. Again, this is not about being sloppy or careless. Your job is to figure out which steps can be skipped.

If you don't understand this about yourself, it can be easy to shut down your creative energy, and play it "safe" with your decisions and choices.

This level of playing small can actually shut down your energy and leave you feeling like your life is mediocre or you may even feel burned out.

STRATEGY: WAIT TO RESPOND AND INFORM

Each Type has a unique Strategy. Strategy is a way of being in the world that begins the process of helping you move from the Conditioned Expression of your energy, to the baseline of your energy. As a Time Bender, you have an inner compass called your Sacral that lets you know when an opportunity feels right. You're designed to follow what feels good, but sometimes Time Benders have to re-learn how to trust that inner feeling.

Your logical mind, and cultural conditioning may have trained you to ignore this vital inner compass. Your Sacral works best when you wait to see what shows up in your life, and then allow yourself to follow the things that feel good. It can feel hard to wait to respond because you've been trained to go out and "make it happen."

If you slow down (which can be very hard!) and wait to see what shows up in your life, and then "feel" your way into it, you will slowly recover your connection to your powerful inner compass. Once something feels good and aligned and your Sacral says "go", you move very quickly, often taking quantum leaps over others.

It's important for the Time Bender, even though it feels unnatural, to take stock of who will be impacted by your choices and make sure you inform them about what you're about to do. Your internal, non-verbal creative flow can cause you to struggle with translating what you're about to do into words. Stopping to explain what you're doing, or that you do not need any help can cause you to lose your connection to your flow. As unnatural as it can seem, when you inform the people who will be impacted by your actions, it can actually prepare the way for you to follow your creative flow with minimal disruption.

Informing isn't asking permission. You don't need permission. Informing simply allows people to move out of your way and support you so you can take action on your inspirations. Your natural alignment with your inner creative flow ultimately benefits everyone around you.

Time Benders have two primary focuses in life: work and family. Time Benders are multi-taskers, oftentimes serial entrepreneurs. You need, and love, to do more than one thing at a time. You often speed through creating anything and everything you consider.

Time Benders respond quickly to situations because of the motor to the Throat, so it's difficult to tell the difference between responding and initiating. Once a response is made, the Time Bender should stop and envision their next decision. You will do well if you visualize outcomes before beginning. You must still wait before taking action.

It is normal and healthy for Time Benders to be starting many projects at the same time. You do not have to complete these projects but instead need to follow the flow of the projects that feel good as they are unfolding in a satisfying way.

This process of trying many things simultaneously often causes others to judge the Time Bender for over-committing, or lack of focus, but this is actually an important part of the creative process of the Time Bender. You need to be free to try many things at once.

EMOTIONAL THEME: ANGER AND FRUSTRATION

We are taught that learning and eventual mastery is a linear process. The more effort you put into it, the more you learn, and the better you get. This just isn't true for you, my dear Time Bender!

You have a stair-step learning curve. When you learn something new, you have an initial surge in mastery. You quickly get good at whatever you're learning. Once you reach a certain level, it's normal for you to sit on a plateau where, no matter how hard you try, you feel stuck and like you're not making any progress.

This is when you feel frustrated, and like the Alchemist, this is when you quit. Frustration may have caused you to be a recurring quitter. Leaping from thing to thing, and trying to find satisfying, meaningful, and fulfilling work to do in the world.

Plateaus are normal for you! The challenge is learning how to work with the frustration that comes with plateaus. Frustration is often a symptom of energy building and momentum gathering for the next surge in mastery. You may have had the experience of waking up, and suddenly finding that your skills improved even though it seems like you didn't do anything to improve them. This is a natural phenomenon for a Time Bender and part of your stair-step learning curve.

Because you're here to find the fastest way to do something, it's normal for you to leap over plateaus and sometimes skip steps. This can also cause you to feel frustrated and angry. Sometimes, you may find that you have to go back and fix the step you skipped.

The second source of frustration in your life can come from feeling like you have tremendous potential, but you don't know how to tap into it. This can be especially true if you've followed all the "rules" of success that your family and society have laid out for you, but you still don't feel like what you've created is meaningful and satisfying. Chronic frustration is an important signal that often lets you know that your life has been constructed from a series of misaligned choices.

You can also experience anger in your life - either from within or from others - when your creative flow gets disrupted. Your anger really isn't what we typically think of as anger as much as it's the result of your creative energy being interrupted. Once you leap into action, you enter an internal non-verbal creative flow. If this flow is interrupted, often by well-meaning people, your energy becomes dissipated because it didn't get to fulfill its purpose. The anger you feel is a symptom of creative disruption.

Other people can also be angry with you when you fail to inform them, and they don't understand what you're doing. It's normal for you to experience anger periodically. If you are experiencing chronic anger in your life, it's important to explore if your natural creative flow is being supported and honored by yourself and those around you.

Time Benders experience deep frustration by initiating (starting) things until they learn how to know the difference between pure inspiration versus the hidden agendas living in their head.

For example, years ago I had an idea for a workshop, after organizing and marketing it like crazy, the sales for the workshop were almost nonexistent! Talk about frustrating! My hidden motivation for pushing this workshop into form was a need for money and a need to prove to myself (and the world) that I wasn't "crazy" for pursuing this alternative career path.

Afterwards, as I started integrating my Time Bender way of being, I waited and waited (the worst!) until someone suggested I teach a workshop about Human Design, giving me something to "respond" to. I responded to that request, and the workshop sold out!

Of course, waiting can feel very challenging. It may feel unnatural for us, particularly in our culture, as we are told to get out there and just do it. Make something happen. If you're a Time Bender, experiment with waiting—try it for just a few days. See what happens! When Time Benders wait, things always come to them at the right time and the right way.

HEALTH

Time Benders also have sustainable life-force energy for doing. You are designed to start with a "full tank of gas" every morning and use up that energy before you go to bed. Although your energy is fast and sustainable, it is not inexhaustible (even though you often think you're inexhaustible!).

Here are some ways that Time Benders can lose energy or burn out. They will experience a variety of "complications" that will wear down their energy:

• Not loving your work environment

• Sedentary lifestyles

• Not following their Sacral guidance (your gut impulses)

• Over-exerting themselves and not recharging their energy

• Feeling chronically frustrated, angry and impatient when results aren't materializing

QUANTUM EXPRESSION:

The masterful Time Bender is aware of their power and speed. They are deeply conscious of those around them, especially those who will be impacted by their responses to life. The masterful Time Bender tunes into the signal of their Sacral Center and waits for something to respond to before leaping into action.

The Time Bender's capacity to "do," changes the story of what can be done in time and on time. The inner alignment of the Time Bender binds them to a creative flow that brings change, transformation, and creativity to the world in new ways. The wisdom of the Time Bender is that, through their experience, they are wise about which steps are necessary to masterfully create and which steps can be skipped.

When responding, the awakened Time Bender has the capacity to bring creative projects to fulfillment, and become masterful over how to work directly with their creative flow and experience of time. Their ability to "do" transforms people's perceptions of what's possible. You are here to remind us that creation can happen instantaneously if we remove our limitations and stay aligned with the unfolding of the Divine Plan.

As our perception of time is evolving, the Time Benders have a unique way of bending and using time. Watch the Time Benders in your life, and you'll witness new ways to use time and flow.

LESSON/CHALLENGE:

To learn to wait for the next right step to inform before acting. To accept that not all actions will result in the success they envision. To recognize the role of the Time Bender is to find the most efficient way to create. To embrace the inner sense of timing, married with action, unique to the energy of the Time Bender, and to follow at their correct speed without self-judgment.

AFFIRMATION:

I move faster than most people. My speed and ability to create many things simultaneously give me a unique perspective on getting things done on the planet. Because I have a lot of energy, I need a lot of movement to stay healthy and strong. It's healthy for me to multitask; I need to do more than one thing at a time to move my energy. Not everything that I do will create the result that I'm envisioning. The purpose of multitasking is to burn off my extra energy. The things that are mine to complete and bring to the world will align with my inner sense of timing, married with action. I am careful to let the people around me know what I'm doing so that they can stand back and let me create at my own speed.

Some famous Time Benders are Frederic Chopin, Marie Curie, Hillary Clinton, Sigmund Freud, Mahatma Gandhi, Marie Antoinette, Mikhail Gorbachev, Jimi Hendrix, Janis Joplin, Friedrich Nietzsche, Richard Nixon, Yoko Ono, Prince, Martin Luther King, Vincent Van Gogh, Malala Yousafzai, and Nicki Minaj.

THE PROJECTOR → ORCHESTRATOR

You are an Orchestrator. Your purpose in life is to manage and guide others toward fulfilling their potential. You have a natural way of knowing the potential of a situation or person, and you instinctively know exactly what needs to be done to create the desired outcome. Your unique knowledge and ability to know what needs to be done is not for everyone. What you know is so precious and valuable. You are designed to share it only with those ready for the transformation you bring.

As an Orchestrator, you are not here to work in the traditional way we define work. You are here to know others, recognize them, direct and guide them, but that can only happen if you are recognized and invited to do so.

Orchestrators, for all your wisdom, can have a frustrating and debilitating life process if you try to push yourself to initiate action. An Orchestrator simply does not have the energy to "just do it." If you try to initiate or work steadily, you will burn yourself out very quickly.

You are a "non-energy" type. You are not here to work steadily like 70% of the population, as an Orchestrator you may receive a lot of judgment from others. You may be perceived as "lazy" when, in fact, it is unhealthy for you to initiate any kind of action, or work, at the wrong kind of job steadily. You usually can't sustain the energy flow on your own. Orchestrators are here to understand others deeply.

Orchestrators can become powerful resources if they are recognized and their guidance is used properly. An Orchestrator can, simply by watching another energy Type, intuitively know how that other person can maximize their energy and their potential. This knowledge makes them natural coaches and mentors. Orchestrators can become the natural managers and leaders of the world.

Orchestrators are highly empathic, sensing the energies of others, and managing them. As an Orchestrator, you have to wait to be recognized and invited into the major events in life, such as love relationships, careers, and the "right place" (where you live.) In between invitations, you should follow your passion and spend your time and energy pursuing your interests and your curiosity.

CONDITIONED EXPRESSION:

As an Orchestrator, you operate like the machine used to project a movie on the wall. You can be in a room surrounded by people who can "see" the vision you're projecting. Still, often, your audience gets distracted from the screen by popcorn, the cute person sitting next to them, or their anticipation for what they will do after the movie.

You may have a lifetime of valiantly trying to get everyone's attention, turning up the volume, and attempting to direct everyone's attention to the screen, but to no avail. It isn't until you're in the right room, at the right time, with people who see your true value - and the value of your vision - that the audience realizes you know exactly how to lead them into bringing the projected vision on the screen into reality.

The biggest challenge for you as an Orchestrator is energy. You don't have a lot of sustainable energy for working in the traditional way we think of as "work." Because of this, you need to structure your life, including how you work, in a way that allows for significant cycles of rest and restoration. Hard work, depleting work mixed with hustle, doesn't serve your purpose, sustainability, or health. To be sustainable and healthy, you must learn how to leverage what you know and the insights and wisdom you bring to any job or relationship.

Orchestrators have a deep energy need for recognition. Being "seen" by the right people allows you to share yourself in a fulfilling and satisfying way. You may find that you compromise your value to be "seen" and recognized. To many Orchestrators, being "seen" and recognized, even if it's for the "wrong" thing, feels better than waiting for people to notice the value that you carry. Ultimately, this can lead to exhaustion, depletion, and burnout.

As an Orchestrator, you must value yourself enough to structure your work so that you are paid for your ideas, insights, and consulting. It's easy for you to give your intellectual property and wisdom away (for free) in the hopes that it will "buy" you the desired recognition. Giving free samples can also exhaust and deplete you and lead to burnout.

Orchestrators struggle with being heard or having ideas stolen. It's counterintuitive, but learning to wait until someone asks you is often the most profitable strategy for the Orchestrator. It makes for an interesting way to do business and life.

You may find it takes a lot of courage to trust the process, and stop pushing and fighting to be seen. Once you realize that your energy can attract the right people, you learn to "call in" the right circumstances simply by valuing yourself and waiting to see who responds to your energy.

When things don't go as planned, or the recognition feels slow in coming, the Orchestrators can experience bitterness. Managing bitterness is crucial because it can repel people instead of attracting them if it is not kept in check. This management takes a lot of self-mastery, patience, and trust in the abundance of the Universe.

Suppose an invitation feels good for you as an Orchestrator and is accepted. In that case, an enormous amount of energy and power is channeled into that situation, which you may use to manage others and the world.

The challenge for the Orchestrator is to trust that the right invitations will come to you and to wait for those invitations. Sometimes, Orchestrators wait months or years for the right invitation, but you can influence the speed and the timing.

To influence the speed at which you can receive invitations, they need two things:

- The energy to implement the invitation

- The Self-Worth to wait for the invitation that is truly honoring of their gifts and talents

Compromising on these two factors can lead to burnout and, often, the emotional theme of bitterness.

Most people don't like to be given advice or told what to do if they haven't first asked for that advice or guidance. Orchestrators who are not using their energy—and their inherent wisdom— correctly are often perceived as:

- Pushy

- Bossy

- Nosy

- Annoying or irritating

- Bitter

The Orchestrator will be ignored and literally not heard when they speak. This lack of being heard and seen can sometimes lead to feeling lonely, misunderstood, and bitter. Orchestrators who use their energy CORRECTLY are respected and sought-after for their knowledge, talent, and guidance.

In addition, because very few Orchestrators learn how to access energy properly, they often face the greatest challenges of all Types when it comes to abundance. In a world that equates money with hard work, it is challenging for Orchestrators to value their wisdom and contribution more than their labor. Because of this, you must build a healthy reserve fund to support yourself during cycles of rest and renewal. This reserve fund will keep you from having to make desperate financial decisions when you're feeling depleted and exhausted.

STRATEGY: WAIT FOR THE INVITATION AND RECOGNITION

Each Type has a unique Strategy, a way of being in the world that begins the process of helping you move from the Conditioned Expression of your energy to the Baseline of your energy.

As an Orchestrator, the most important thing you can do to protect your energy is to wait for the right people who see your vision and value to recognize and invite you to share your guidance. You're here to be seen and invited into the big opportunities of life, such as relationships, work, or moving to a new place. Those invitations usually only come once a year or so.

While waiting, you get to do whatever you want, provided you are honoring yourself and have the energy for it. While you're waiting for life's big invitations, sustaining yourself by nurturing and caring for your energy is vital.

The in-between time is a great time to pursue your passions and explore what interests and intrigues you. You may find your next invitation involves what you've been learning and exploring while you were waiting.

Orchestrators fear they will not be invited. However, if you follow your strategy of waiting for the invitation, your aura's frequency starts to change. The more you live according to your design, the more invitations you get. Living by your design will bring you SUCCESS.

Once invited, you don't need to wait for further invitations regarding whatever you were invited to (project, job, relationship, etc.). Just wait for the right people and the right invitation, and the rest will click into place. The invitation, the correct entry into anything, is the key.

If the feeling of being recognized, appreciated, heard, and seen is there, you're in the right place with the right people. If not, you may stop talking mid-sentence and save yourself the disappointment of not being understood.

While the natural role (and instinct) of the Orchestrator is to "manage, guide and direct others," the Orchestrator can only do so effectively when others want to be managed, guided, and directed!

Orchestrators are the eternal students of humanity and system masters. You need to have a system through which you can relate and understand life. The BEST approach for an Orchestrator is to wait to be asked or invited before sharing their advice, opinion, feedback, guidance, or direction.

When someone asks, it is an indication they want the guidance and inherent wisdom of that Orchestrator. (Even if that person is completely unaware that they are asking an Orchestrator, that person is unconsciously reacting to the Orchestrator's energetic configuration). That person will then hear and appreciate the value of the Orchestrator's input because they were open to receiving it.

The NEXT BEST approach for the Orchestrator is to at least wait for some recognition and an opening to speak. Make eye contact and wait to sense an opportunity to speak without barging into a conversation or seeming pushy or overbearing.

When using this NEXT BEST approach, the most effective way for an Orchestrator to begin is to say something like:

- I have some experience that may be helpful to you. Would it be all right if I shared it with you?

- I have some insights about that. May I tell you more about them?

- Perhaps I could be of help. Would you mind if I tried?

You still may not get the response that is a clear invitation, but this at least gives the Orchestrator a tiny opening to moving their powerful wisdom out into the world.

EMOTIONAL THEME: BITTERNESS

Bitterness is a repelling energy. You might struggle to see the brilliance of feeling bitter until you realize that bitterness is your signal that you're out of energy. When your emotional theme "repels" people, it's because you're not ready for an invitation just yet. You probably don't have the energy for a new opportunity, or you're about to take an invitation that doesn't reflect your value.

Energy is of premium importance for an Orchestrator. You don't have the same reserves of energy as others. In short bursts, you have more energy than everyone else, but eventually, you may find you hit a wall and feel exhausted and depleted.

Most Orchestrators are well-trained to push against depletion. There is no way to regain your energy other than resting and renewing yourself. When you feel bitter, you push people away because you lack the energy for invitations. Rest and play, then you'll find you are, once again, hopeful and energized.

Sometimes, Orchestrators have to heal their self-worth to give themselves permission to rest without guilt or shame. You need to sustain yourself to better serve others. You're not like most people. Your contribution to the world isn't necessarily about doing the grunt work.

You're a leader who is here to help people fulfill their purpose by guiding those who are ready for you. Don't compromise and settle for trying to guide people who don't see your value.

You're a leader who is here to help people fulfill their purpose by guiding those who are ready for you. Don't compromise and settle for trying to guide people who don't see your value. Bitterness is a clear signal that you need to pull back, replenish your energy, and work on healing your self-worth so that you only accept recognition and attention from people aligned with your vision and values.

HEALTH

Pushing and forcing will never have a positive outcome for Orchestrators. Pushing and forcing will always have the opposite effect and lead to burnout. The more you attempt to push, force, or struggle your way into being "seen" or recognized, the more invisible (and bitter) you become.

Not only that, Orchestrators have a very finite amount of energy and are not meant to work in the traditional way work is designed. You will burn out if pushed into situations where you aren't recognized for your inherent, intuitive gifts or that is hard physical labor.

Orchestrators can't make life work for them if they follow the standard definitions of what it takes to succeed, although Orchestrators can be powerful and very successful. (For example, President Obama and President Kennedy are both Orchestrators).

When Orchestrators push or force, they push people away rather than attract them. Because working hard isn't an option for the limited energy of the Orchestrator, no matter how hard they try, the Orchestrator can often feel that life isn't "fair" and become bitter.

Getting good, healthy sleep is of particular importance for you, and to do so, you need to lie down before you feel tired. You can read or watch a movie for a while before you fall asleep, but do so while lying in a horizontal position. Being flat in a horizontal position allows you to release the energy you've taken during the day and helps your body discharge excess energy. Your sensitivity can be energetically exhausting, so having your own space to relax is important. Learning to say "no" and permitting yourself to rest is vital to sustaining your health.

QUANTUM EXPRESSION:

The awakened Orchestrator nurtures and cares for their mind, body, and Spirit with great deliberation. They understand that timing and waiting are forces that work in their favor, and they use the time between activations to rest and restore their energy.

An awakened Orchestrator knows their value, and they stand in their value with the awareness that what they have to give will only serve its purpose if they share it with the right people at the right time. They recognize that timing is not about their personal value but about the readiness and timing of the opportunity. They trust in the right timing and understand the right opportunity will reveal itself when the timing is right, and the value is correctly placed.

The awakened Orchestrator knows that they are here to deliver knowledge and wisdom; not necessarily do the work of creating the physical form of the creation. They allow others to do the work while managing, guiding, and delegating to conserve and use their energy effectively. Orchestrators truly serve as the "midwives" of the future.

You have a deep inner sense of what's possible for the world and know how to direct the necessary energy to bring the non-tangible into form.

You are an energy wizard and are, on an unconscious level, constantly realigning and managing the world's energy flow. This work goes way beyond the tangible physical work of the Sacral Types who have the workforce energy. This work is energy, and the Orchestrator keeps the energy grid of creation in place.

Orchestrators often report being "tired all the time" even when they do "nothing." An Orchestrator never does "nothing." You are in a constant state of holding together the world's energy grid. Because Orchestrators know energy so well, they are often involved in energy healing and service-based professions. You are a natural healer and helper.

LESSON/CHALLENGE:

The lesson of the Orchestrator is to learn to value themselves and their wisdom enough to wait for the right opportunity to share their knowledge and insights. To facilitate the correct experiences that reflect their value, the Orchestrator needs to maintain a high sense of self-worth and cultivate their energy by resting and replenishing themselves to be sustainable.

AFFIRMATION:

I am a powerful resource for the world. My intuition, insights, awareness, and knowledge helps manage and guide the energy of the world and the next phase of growth and evolution on the planet. What I offer the world is so powerful, necessary, and valuable that I recognize I am carrying the seeds of evolution within my being. I wait for the right opportunities that reflect the value of what I carry and bring into the world. When the opportunity is correct and I am valued, I share my knowledge and wisdom and facilitate the work necessary to build the next phase of the human story. In between opportunities, I rest and replenish my energy to be ready to serve when I am called again.

Other famous Orchestrators include Taylor Swift, Esther Hicks, Barack Obama, Nelson Mandela, Queen Elizabeth II, Mick Jagger, Barbara Streisand, Liz Taylor, Lance Armstrong, Abraham Lincoln, James Joyce, Brad Pitt, John F. Kennedy, Karl Marx, and Marilyn Monroe.

THE REFLECTOR → CALIBRATOR

You are a Calibrator, a rare Quantum Human Design Type!

You're here to embody and reflect back to the world the quality of the energy surrounding you. You feel happy if you're in a happy place with happy people.

If you're in an unhappy place with unhappy people, you can feel unhappy until you learn to regulate your energy. Your ability to sense, feel, and know the energy around you makes you a barometer for others to gauge the health of the shared community environment.

As you mature, and get to know how your energy works better, you'll learn how to be at home within yourself, and even though you will still experience and know your outer environment, you won't identify with it the way you might now. You'll realize that you can be at home in any place as you learn to regulate your internal environment and energy.

Calibrators are fully open to the world and others. You take in everybody else's energy, seeing the world through others' eyes, sampling a frequency of energy, and reflecting it back to the other. You are like a mirror, and the reflection of other people continually changes their perception.

You may feel extremely emotional in one instant, while the next moment, it's gone. You may then get all the ideas and a sound sense of knowing where you're going in life, and then it's gone again, and so forth. That's why it's essential for you to carefully choose your friends and partners. They will have a tremendous impact on your feelings and experience of yourself.

Your purpose in life is to be the "barometer" of the health of the community around you and to also, through your own embodiment, quietly live out the highest expression of the human story.

People look to you to see what's possible. There is no outer work associated with this purpose. It is simply fulfilling what you know is possible for humanity with clear intention and integrity. You are here to show the world what justice, peace, abundance, and compassion look like. When you embody these archetypes, you lift up the energy around you simply by being yourself.

63

Calibrators have considerably unique life experiences compared to the other Types. Because of this, sometimes you may feel alone and misunderstood. Calibrators can also suffer deep disappointment when having to wait and live through the energy of others. Sometimes, you may feel inadequate and think you don't fit anywhere.

The most uncomfortable thing for Calibrators is pressure, especially the pressure to make decisions quickly. To make good, clear choices, you need time to "feel" your way through your decisions. In a fast-paced world, it can often feel like you're being pressured to decide before you feel ready.

As a Calibrator, you reflect the energy of those surrounding you, enmeshed and embedded in the personal stories of others, until you realize your experience of the energy can reveal other options to others. In the experience of the world around you, co-mingled with the wisdom of your understanding of the potential that comes from such profound empathy, you can learn to use your energy to reveal to the world how the reflection needs to be better calibrated towards growth and expansion.

Because of your sensitivity to others and how you can sometimes confuse your own energy with the energy of others, you must wait 29 days before making any major decisions - no matter how certain you feel about something at the moment.

As a Calibrator, it often helps at the beginning of learning about your energy to be in the right geographical location, the place that feels good and like "home" for your life to feel "right." When you are in the right place, you meet the right people, you are part of the right community, and your life feels aligned. Under these circumstances, making decisions can feel easier and less disappointing.

The more you are in a place that feels "right," the more you learn to internalize this feeling and, ultimately, learn to make a part of your inner sense of being "at home" within yourself. You learn to stay connected to integrity and alignment no matter what happens around you.

Calibrators often struggle with "merging" in their personal relationships if they don't understand the nature of their sensitivity and their capacity for deep empathy. Sometimes, your energy can get "hijacked" by the energy of the people surrounding you, and you can lose your own direction in life.

It's easy for you to fall in love with people's potential and get confused by the energy you're experiencing. Your energy always changes depending on who you're with and where you are. Because of this, you like to be around people you know and whose energy feels familiar to you. This familiarity means sometimes making changes or healthier choices is extra hard because you often have to give up the known and consistent things to break away and create change. You need time to really sense your own energy in the intensity of all the energy you absorb and reflect.

Consistency is vital for the Calibrator. You need to have people whose aura you know. It is common for you to have lifelong friends and even have trouble disentangling yourself from the energy of your parents (your family of origin) simply because your experience is so inconsistent that clinging to people you know feels comforting. The consistency of the people you know makes you feel safe but can sometimes keep you "stuck" in relationships or situations you've outgrown.

As a Calibrator, it might take some time to make the necessary changes to reflect your personal growth and evolution. Because you need time for clarity and to make decisions, you don't transition quickly and need time for clarity and to make decisions, and you don't transition quickly and need time to make major life changes, such as leaving home, moving, starting a new job, or even getting married. The pressure to "hurry up" can sometimes cause you to leap into decisions because of the pressure and then feel deeply disappointed in the outcome of your choice.

STRATEGY: WAIT A LUNAR CYCLE (IN OTHER WORDS, TAKE YOUR TIME!)

Each Type has a unique Strategy, a way of being in the world that begins the process of helping you move from the Conditioned Expression of your energy to the Baseline of your energy.

As a Calibrator, you have a strategy that is intricately interwoven with the movement of the moon and your need for time for clarity. You are not here to be spontaneous. Your chart changes daily with the moon's movement and with your experience of the world around you.

You need time to connect with yourself and find the thread of your authentic needs, wants, and desires amid all the energy you process. It can often be one or more full lunar cycles before you have clarity around your choices.

You may find it helps to talk out your current thoughts and ideas for the day. You don't need advice from others, just a sounding board to hear your thoughts and feelings out loud. Externally processing through speech helps you know yourself and your current feelings better. Take your time to decide on the big things in life. You deserve it!

Calibrators must know and logically understand any kind of pressure you experience is detrimental to your health. By taking the time to make important decisions and understanding the time spent considering your choices is what completes your success, you will realize how vital it is to avoid letting anyone pressure you. You experience a choice or decision over a cycle of the moon (29 days). It's not the same as deciding with the mind. Calibrators have to experience their choices inside of themselves over time. Going through the entire cycle gives you the power to realize solutions and make the right choices for yourself.

Calibrators are lunar beings tied to the lunar cycle, so your Strategy (and sometimes the challenge) is to wait 29 days before making any major decisions. During the 29 days, Calibrators should talk with different people about decisions. As a Calibrator, you need to have people in your life who will serve as your sounding board, not because you need advice (you don't), but because you need to hear yourself talk about what you are feeling about your choices.

Life for you is an objective experience. As you move through life, discover the truth of "this isn't me" over and over again. Your sensitivity may be energetically exhausting, so having your own space to relax is important. The same goes for rest and sleep. The Calibrator needs to go to bed as soon as you begin to feel tired and, if possible, sleep alone.

Calibrators / Reflectors carry a deep potential to know the possibilities for humanity in their being. This potential can be a beautiful thing.

EMOTIONAL THEME: DISAPPOINTMENT

As a Calibrator, you take in and experience a wide variety of human energies. Over time, you see the potential for all of humanity, and you can often feel disappointed in humanity. Therefore, you often crave being with children, animals, and joyful people who have done their inner work. It feels better to surround yourself with people who are healthy and have done the inner work to activate their potential.

You can also feel disappointed with yourself for making the "wrong" choice due to feeling pressured to make fast decisions. We live in a very fast-paced world. It's hard to make a big decision, such as buying a car, or deciding which college scholarship you should accept, without feeling pressured to decide quickly. This pressure can sometimes cause you to make choices without taking the necessary time to decide in a way that's aligned with your energy. Do your best to take as much time as you need - especially for big decisions!

Calibrators have the capacity to sense, feel, and know the full potential of the people and the communities around them. Your Openness gives you deep awareness and wisdom about what is possible for the world.

It is disappointing for the Calibrator to know what's possible and see the world isn't fulfilling its full potential. Disappointment also comes because of the speed of the world. The Calibrator's need for ample time to make clear, and good decisions doesn't always match with the pace of the world.

When a Calibrator fails to take their time in deciding and struggles to find their own energy amid the energy they are experiencing from others, it's easy for a Calibrator to feel pressured into making a choice quickly. (And, collectively, we have little patience for people who need time for clarity.) Consequently, Calibrators can leap into decisions too quickly and then feel disappointed with the long-term consequences of their decisions.

HEALTH

There are three major factors to staying healthy if you are a Calibrator:

- You need to be in an environment that feels good to you, and the people in your environment need to be healthy. Because you are so sensitive to others and the experience of others, if you are in an environment where people aren't making healthy choices, that will deeply impact you. As you move from the Calibrator Baseline of your Type to fully living as a Calibrator, this need can shift as you learn to be "at home" within yourself.

- You need good sleep and rest. Calibrators sleep best alone and need to be in the energy of their own aura at night to stay vital and replenish their energy. Calibrators must be in bed before they are tired and rest in a prone position until they fall asleep.

- You need to take your time to make the right decisions for you. If you feel pressured to decide before you're ready, it may end up being the wrong choice, and the pressure and struggle to try to feel pressured to decide before you're ready, it may end up being the wrong choice, and the pressure and struggle to try to feel "right" about the decision can deeply impact your physical and emotional health.

Not following through on all three key factors often results in burnout, depletion, and exhaustion.

QUANTUM EXPRESSION:

The awakened Calibrator is aware of their surroundings and the experience of the energy of their surroundings within them. They feel in alignment with their community and within themselves. They experience the people they surround themselves with and the environment they place themselves in as "home."

The awakened Calibrator knows the impact of the energy of others and values themselves enough to take the time to find the alignment with what is right for themselves amid the experience of the energies of so many other people. They are aware of the reflection and can simply "be" with the reflection. They are witnesses, and the power of what they see and reflect is the purpose of their lives.

Despite recognizing the potential, the Calibrator's role is not to fix what isn't working but merely to reflect it back to the community. Calibrators are here to be our Karmic Mirrors. Your life experience and your reflection on us reveal where we are in our evolutionary process. The Calibrators in our lives show us how close we are to fulfilling our potential. They let us know the emotional maturity and alignment we are experiencing by living it and demonstrating it in their own reflected experience. The heart of the Calibrator carries within it the potential for our optimal evolution and the story of what else is possible for humanity.

LESSON/CHALLENGE:

The lesson of the Calibrator is to learn to let go of the need to fix what isn't working, to share and experience what they see and feel, and to trust the Universal flow of right timing will support the world in doing the transformation necessary to create alignment and peace. Calibrators have the job of embodying what they feel, and sense, and using their lives as a mirror of awakening for others, but to remember it is not the job of the Calibrator to do the work of fixing others.

AFFIRMATION:

I am a karmic mirror. Through my experience and expression of the energy around me, I reflect back to others their potential and their misalignment. Through my reflection, others can see what they need to bring back into alignment to fulfill their path. I understand the depth of the potential of possibility for humanity. I know it is not my job to fix the world but to simply mirror the current energies. I trust in Divine Timing, and I know that with time, the potential of the world will be fulfilled. I am patient and honor myself. I give myself the time I need to make the right choices and to place myself in the right location with the right people. I trust my inner sense of feeling at home where I belong and stay aligned with where I feel most at home.

Famous Calibrators include Sandra Bullock, Uri Geller, and Roslyn Carter.

In every story, the main character has to make decisions that drive their evolution. Learning to make effective decisions is a key aspect of reclaiming sovereignty over your life. The Strategy for your Quantum Human Design Type gives you a lot of information about how you can recover and heal your decision-making ability.

Your body is an essential part of your decision-making *Storytelling* process. When presented with an opportunity, the visceral response within the body, gives us key insights into what is truly right for us. Most of us are well-trained to make decisions with our minds. This pattern of thinking our way through our decisions means we have silenced our connection to our body and our bodies' wisdom.

If you disconnect from your body, you leave yourself vulnerable to not only missing vital information for a better life, eventually, your body will experience significant symptoms to get your attention.

Your Authority, listed on your Quantum Human Design chart, shows you what you need to pay attention to, in order to reconnect with the wisdom of your body's messages. Authority helps you remember what it your body has been trying to tell you, and what it will feel like within the body. Although decision-making is tied directly to your Type and Strategy, your Authority shapes the way you use your Strategy.

Your Defined Centers will determine your Authority. Not all centers carry Authority, so your personal Authority will depend on your Type and Definition. The way in which you experience your Authority, will also depend on your life conditioning and your level of emotional well-being.

When you receive a Human Design reading, you are taught to understand patterns of pain, and behaviors that may keep you from living out the beauty of your true story. With cognitive awareness of old patterns, you begin to heal and transform these energies into deep sources of wisdom. The more you clear your old energy patterns, the more effectively your natural decision-making skills (your Authority) can function.

It's very important to note that Authority does not override your Strategy. It just shifts the way you use your strategy. Your decisions and choices more deeply align with the overall energy in your Design. Authority can influence what you need to use your Strategy effectively. For example, an Alchemist with Sacral Authority needs to use their Strategy of waiting to respond. When an opportunity presents itself to the Alchemist, they wait for their inner Sacral Response to give a clear "yes" or "no."

All Generator Types (if they have an undefined Emotional Solar Plexus) have Sacral Authority, called Evolutionary Authority in Quantum Human Design™.

When you have Sacral Authority, it means your gut response in the moment lets you know whether something is right for you or not.

The biggest challenge with Evolutionary Authority is learning to trust your instinctual response. Please read the Alchemist and Time Bender sections to learn more about Evolutionary Authority.

QUANTUM EXPRESSION

The gut-level pulse of Evolutionary Authority informs the Alchemists and the Time Benders about what needs to be done to further the Divine Imperative, and the evolution of the world. Initiators, Orchestrators, Alchemists, Time Benders all have Authority in their Design. Calibrators, because they have no Centers defined in their Design, have no true Authority other than their Calibrator Strategy, which is to wait for a full Lunar cycle.

In the name of keeping it simple, there are four other basic kinds of Authority:

1. Actualizing Authority / Splenic Authority

2. Creative Authority / Emotional Authority

3. Orchestrated Authority / Self Authority

4. Resource Authority / Ego Authority

Different Human Design software programs will list other kinds of Authority, but these variations are simply sub-categories of the 5 basic kinds of Authority.

ACTUALIZING AUTHORITY

Actualizing Authority means you are designed to know, in the moment, what feels right, or wrong, to you. Having Actualizing Authority means you can be spontaneous with your decisions. You don't need time to contemplate or sit with decisions. You will know what is true for you immediately.

Much like Evolutionary Authority, Actualizing Authority is a gut-level sense of what feels right or aligned. For those of you who are not Evolutionary Types, Actualizing Authority can help you make smaller decisions about your daily life choices.

For example, suppose you have Actualizing Authority and are searching for a vitamin supplement at the health food store. In that case, your Self-Actualization Center might give you a "sense" of which vitamin is right for you.

Often, we master Actualizing Authority in hindsight. Actualizing Authority is the feeling of "knowing" something is right, or wrong, and upon later reflection, understanding, you should have listened to yourself. With practice, you can begin to notice your Actualizing Authority at the moment, allowing the wisdom and awareness of your intuition to guide you and give you essential insights about what you need.

QUANTUM DEFINITION

The instinctual awareness to know when it is time to expand resources, align with greater integrity, take actions to sustain or increase value or your own value, and fully self-actualize your gifts, experiences and talents.

CREATIVE AUTHORITY

If you have Creative Authority, you are not designed to be spontaneous. You need time to make decisions, and learning how to wait for clarity is essential to help you not experience disappointment in your life's choices.

Creative Authority can influence the way your Strategy for your Type works. Your Strategy for your Type is still essential, but if you have Creative Authority, it means you have to check in with your Strategy, and "sense" how you feel over time. You tend to have a lot of emotional energy when you have Creative Authority. You are passionate and experience big feelings to various degrees depending on other aspects of your chart.

This internal emotional energy makes it essential you take your time to make decisions. It's easy to leap into things in the moment when they feel good; only to wake up the next day doubting whether you made the right choice. Waiting for clarity helps avoid some of the regrets you may have experienced in your life. With Creative Authority, your decision has to stay consistent over time. If you are all over the place with how you feel about your choice while waiting for clarity, it's probably not the right decision to make.

Here's how this might look. Let's say you get invited to speak at an event sponsored by a group you like but are not crazy about. You love speaking, but you don't necessarily enjoy this particular group. When you get the invitation, you're so excited to land a speaking gig that you immediately accept it. The next morning, when you wake up, you question your decision, and you have a small anxiety stomachache from worrying about whether you did the right thing.

Over the next couple of days, you try to convince yourself it was the right choice. You manage to stir up enthusiasm along the way, but you can't quite get your energy aligned with the opportunity. When you finally give the talk, several group members want to hire you, but they end up being clients you don't enjoy, and you're left continuing to feel obligated to do business in a way that doesn't feel good to you.

If you had followed your Creative Authority when you got invited to speak, you might have answered, "Thank you. This opportunity sounds like a lovely invitation. I need to check my calendar and get back to you. When do you need to know my response?" Your answer would have bought you time to check in with your feelings to see if this was the right choice for you, and you would have been aligned with whatever felt correct.

The most important thing to remember with Creative Authority is your decision has to stay consistent over time. Suppose you feel a "yes" in response to an opportunity. The "yes" has to stay true over a period of time. If you're all over the place with your feelings, it's not the right decision for you.

QUANTUM DEFINITION

The ability to consciously cultivate a baseline emotional frequency that allows you to sense through feeling the right timing and alignment for decisions and actions.

ORCHESTRATED AUTHORITY

This Authority is kind of a catch-all phrase for a few different, less common Authorities. If you have a chart that says Self-Projected

Authority, No Authority, No Inner Authority, or Mental-Projected Authority, it simply means you must talk through your choices to get clarity.

You don't need advice. You need a sounding board, a good friend, or someone you trust who can listen to you while you discuss your options. Having this kind of Authority means that you are gifted at seeking the potential of all possibilities. Talking through the potentials helps you gauge where the energy flows, the conditions field, and your own alignment with what needs to happen to fulfill the potential in your life.

Orchestrated Authority is common for Orchestrator Types and all Calibrators.

QUANTUM DEFINITION

The ability to see the potential in all choices which requires externalization in order to clarify which potential is correct and aligned with action.

RESOURCE AUTHORITY

Having this Authority means you have a defined Resource Center and you don't have Creative Authority. The Resource Center is about having sustainable energy and resources. If you have Resource Authority, you won't decide to do something unless you have the energy or the resources. It also can signal whether a choice is aligned with integrity or not.

This type of Authority can present a challenge because it means you have to have healthy self-worth in order to be comfortable saying "no" to something if you don't have the energy, resources for it or if something about the decision feels out of integrity.

If you're in a pattern of trying to prove your worth by pleasing others, you may find you have to strengthen your sense of value before you can truly follow the Authority of your Resource Center.

QUANTUM DEFINITION

The ability to know when a choice is in alignment with available resources, sustainability, and integrity.

CONCLUSION

Your Quantum Human Design Strategy for your Type, and your Authority, gives you a prescription for remembering the wisdom of your body and how to interpret the messages your body is giving you. This reconnection can help you better tune in to what is right for you so you begin to make choices in a way that is more aligned with your authentic self. The more you relearn to trust the wisdom of your body and how it communicates, the more you begin to create a life that supports your optimal vitality, wellness and well-being - choice by choice by choice.

In this final section, you're going to explore for yourself how to apply the Quantum Alignment System (QAS) to your own story. Using the awareness you've just gained from learning about the "main character" in your story, you're going to explore where, and how you may be holding yourself back from the bold, authentic expression of the person you were born to become, and how you can begin to reclaim the true story of who you really are.

The Quantum Alignment System gives you a systematic and integrated approach to reclaiming your true story. Included in this chapter is a QAS Alignment Protocol for each Type.

Each Protocol contains the following sections:

1. SELF-ASSESSMENT AND CONTEMPLATIONS

In the Self-Assessment section, you will be invited to rate yourself on key themes associated with your Type on a scale of 1-10. A low score indicates you are currently living a story that embodies a conditioned expression of your personal story. A high score indicates you are embodying the optimal expression of your personal story. The goal of this rating is to get you moving up the scale to greater states of vitality, joy and authentic self-expression.

The self-assessment is not designed from a place of judgment. The assessment doesn't indicate you are doing something "wrong" or failing in some way. You need an honest awareness of what you need to shift, and align in your personal story. Remember, with awareness, you have the power to write your story the way YOU choose.

Included in this Self-Assessment step are contemplations to help you explore more of what you may want to rewrite in your personal narrative.

2. A PRIMARY EMOTIONAL FREEDOM TECHNIQUE (EFT)

An EFT setup to get you started with tapping. If you need instructions on how to use EFT, please download our *EFT for Everyone Guide* from the Reader Resource page.

3. A PROPRIETARY QUANTUM QUESTION

We are profoundly conditioned to use our minds to "figure out" our challenges. When we use our minds to try to figure things out, we are usually choosing solutions from the same set of repeated options. We do this because when we are dealing with our story, strictly on the manifestation level, and we're still living from a story that is inauthentic, it's hard for us to clearly see what else is possible.

We are hardwired to tap into the Quantum Field by asking open-ended questions and then waiting to see what catches our attention. What insights "drop" in? Even what we dream about in response to these questions can be important. The Quantum Question process simply gives you a template to ask powerful questions, so you can activate and attract the answers into your physical world.

It is important to understand that you don't - and shouldn't - try to figure out the answers to these questions. It's your job to ask the questions, keep your energy in an optimistic state, and then see what answers show up. The more you work this process, the more you'll see the "magic" in asking, and then receiving the insights, potentials, and answers you're seeking.

Read your Quantum Question before you exercise, go for a walk, before you go to sleep at night, or anytime you start to feel anxious about the challenge you may be facing.

If you want to give yourself a really beautiful pause in your day, listen to the Vitality Synchronizing Sound Frequency and meditate and breathe for a couple of minutes while you silently ask your Quantum Question.

The format for the Quantum Question is:

What needs to be healed, released, aligned, and brought to my awareness for me to _____

____(fill in the end results you're seeking here)?

4. A STORYLAB PROMPT TO HELP YOU START THE PROCESS OF REWRITING YOUR PERSONAL STORY.

We know from science that the act of writing a story refocuses our attention, programs the brain to find external evidence that the story is already coming true, improves some gene functions, increases your immune response, and can make you more resilient and creative. In this section, you will be given a list of story prompts, contemplations, and a "story specimen" that will help you use intentional storytelling to rewrite your story.

This process, called StoryLab, may take you an hour or two. Give yourself the gift of time so you can focus on this deeply moving process that will not only give you a different perspective on your story but can help you find your true voice to tell the story of who you are YOUR way.

5. A CUSTOMIZED SYNCHRONIZING SOUND FREQUENCY TUNED TO THE FREQUENCY OF VITALITY

Once you feel complete with your story, use the Synchronizing Sound Frequency (the link can be found on the Reader Resource page) to tune into your new story.

This process will require about 10 minutes of your time. Make sure you have privacy and an uninterrupted space to complete this part of the process.

When you're ready, take 10 minutes for yourself. Close the door. Relax. Read your new story to yourself and focus on where you feel your new story in your body. Put your hand over this place to help you remember what this level of alignment feels like in your body. When you feel ready, using a good set of headphones, listen to the synchronizing frequency at normal volume and enjoy your attunement!

INITIATOR / MANIFESTOR:

1. SELF ASSESSMENT AND CONTEMPLATIONS:

Think about your energy. Contemplate whether you feel vital or whether you feel burned out. Take a moment and rank how vital you feel from 0-10

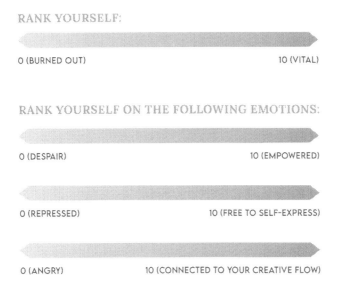

RANK YOURSELF:

0 (BURNED OUT)   10 (VITAL)

RANK YOURSELF ON THE FOLLOWING EMOTIONS:

0 (DESPAIR)   10 (EMPOWERED)

0 (REPRESSED)   10 (FREE TO SELF-EXPRESS)

0 (ANGRY)   10 (CONNECTED TO YOUR CREATIVE FLOW)

CONTEMPLATIONS:

- How do you feel about being powerful?
- Were you allowed to "follow your own flow" as a child?
- Was your power acknowledged and supported by those around you?
- Do you feel comfortable being powerful?
- Is anger a theme in your life?
- Does your fear of anger or your suppression of anger stop you from doing what you want in life?
- What needs to be healed, released, aligned, and brought to your awareness for you to fully embrace the value of your unique initiating role in the world?

- Are you out of physical, moral, resource, identity, or energetic integrity?
- What do you need to do to be in integrity with yourself, your energy, or others?
- What needs to be healed, released, aligned, and brought to your awareness for you to trust
your own powerful connection to your own right timing?

2. PRIMARY EFT SETUP:

- Even though I'm afraid to fully express my power, I deeply and completely love and accept myself.
- Even though I don't trust my connection to my creative flow, I deeply and completely love and accept myself.

3. QUANTUM QUESTION:

What needs to be released, healed, aligned and brought to my awareness for me to fully express my power?

Flower Essences: Quantum Alignment System Initiator/Manifestor Formula

4. STORYLAB PROMPT:

STORY SPECIMEN: THE MANIFESTOR

She had a reputation for doing her own thing and being "emotional" when she didn't get her way. This didn't always translate well in her relationships.

Her parents were constantly frustrated with her, judging her and scolding her for her temper and for being impulsive. She was often punished harshly and learned quickly how to hide her emotions and her desires in order to stay safe and avoid feeling overpowered. She always felt like others were watching to see what she was "up to" so she learned to get better at hiding as she got older.

Eventually, she hid so well that she forgot her power. She learned to suppress her anger and her creative urges. She learned to "play the game," to fit in, and to use her energy to be "good." But deep inside, she knew it wasn't right. She could feel her inner self calling her out, begging her to follow her creative instincts. Inside of her was a rich, inspired world. A world that spoke to her in flashes of inspiration and insight, and begged her to follow these vital prompts. She couldn't explain it to others. It was almost a primal, powerful voice that pulled at her as she followed her daily routines.

The louder the voice got, the more uncomfortable her life became. She began to realize she'd abdicated her power in every area of her life - her work, her relationships - even in the way she nurtured herself. She was exhausted and depleted from trying to hold it together and deny this powerful voice inside of her.

She realized she needed to break free...

What comes next in the story? How do you want to write the ending of this story in such a way that it inspires you, lifts you up, and encourages you to continue to reclaim your authentic story in your everyday life?

Do you relate to this specimen? Which parts?

Write your new story starting with the following template:

Once upon a time, there was a _____ (your main character description goes here).

Until one day _____
_____ (What cataclysmic event or experience causes your main character to "wake up" to the true story of who you are? This can be fantastical, realistic, rooted in your real-life experiences or as wild and bold as you choose.)

Until she _____
_____ (What does your main character learn or realize? What lessons and blessings does she learn to bring to others? How does she embody her new understanding and her new gifts?)

Take some time and really savor this creative process.

5. SYNCHRONIZING SOUND FREQUENCY

When you're ready, take 10 minutes for yourself. Close the door. Relax. Read your new story to yourself and really focus on where you feel your new story in your body. Put your hand over this place to help you remember what this level of alignment feels like in your body. When you feel ready, using a good set of headphones, listen to the synchronizing frequency at normal volume and enjoy your personal attunement!

ALCHEMIST / GENERATOR:

1. SELF ASSESSMENT AND CONTEMPLATIONS:

Think about your energy. Contemplate whether you feel vital or whether you feel burned out. Take a moment and rank how vital you feel from 0-10

RANK YOURSELF:

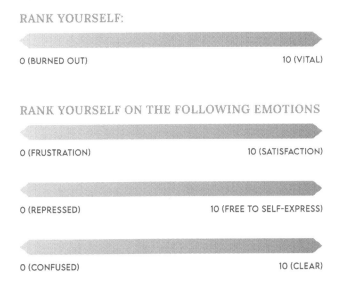

0 (BURNED OUT)　　　　　　　　　　　　　　　　10 (VITAL)

RANK YOURSELF ON THE FOLLOWING EMOTIONS

0 (FRUSTRATION)　　　　　　　　　　　　　10 (SATISFACTION)

0 (REPRESSED)　　　　　　　　　　　10 (FREE TO SELF-EXPRESS)

0 (CONFUSED)　　　　　　　　　　　　　　　10 (CLEAR)

CONTEMPLATIONS:

- How do you experience frustration?
- Where do you feel it in your body?
- What is your habit when you feel frustrated?
- Are you frustrated about your life right now?
- What is your response to your current frustration?
- Do you trust your Sacral?
- Do you trust that your next right step will show up for you?
- How do you feel about waiting?
- What can you do to cultivate more patience and alignment?

2. PRIMARY EFT SETUP:

- Even though my frustration keeps me from fully actualizing anything, I deeply and completely love and accept myself.

- Even though I'm frustrated with the manifestations of my life...

- Even though I'm afraid of getting it wrong...

3. QUANTUM QUESTION:

What needs to be released, healed, aligned, and brought to my awareness for me to fully live a fulfilled and satisfied life?

Flower Essences: Quantum Alignment System Alchemist Formula

4. STORYLAB PROMPT:

STORY SPECIMEN: THE GENERATOR

From the start, she had an inner sense of feeling right and joyful to her. She grunted with delight at the food she loved and the games she liked to play. She also grunted and made faces at the things she didn't like but was quickly told she was rude. And that not using words was unacceptable.

She was told, over and over again, "You don't always get to do what you want to do." She was told, "You must follow the rules and do what is expected of you."

The expectations of:

- Get good grades.

- Get in with the right people.

- Get into the right school.

- Get a successful career.

She learned to disconnect from her body's wisdom and to ignore those inner signals of what felt right or wrong. She learned to make decisions with her mind - doing what seemed logical and reasonable. She learned to follow the rules and do those things the world told her she needed to do to be successful. She settled for a quiet life of mediocrity. She learned to numb her frustration with food and media, telling herself that someday she'd be free to do what lit her up inside.

Sometimes, she tried new things, but she always hit a plateau and felt frustrated. Eventually, she quit. The frustration always made her wonder if life and work were just supposed to be hard and there was no way out until she retired when she could follow her passion and do what she wanted to do.

Until one day, she realized she just couldn't do it anymore...

What comes next in the story? How do you want to write the ending of this story in such a way that it inspires you, lifts you up, and encourages you to continue to reclaim your authentic story in your everyday life?

Do you relate to this specimen? Which parts?

Write your new story starting with the following template:

Once upon a time, there was a _____
_____ (your main character description goes here).

Until one day _____
_____ (What cataclysmic event or experience causes your main character to "wake up" to the true story of who you are? This can be fantastical, realistic, rooted in your real-life experiences or as wild and bold as you choose.)

Until she _____
_____ (What does your main character learn or realize? What lessons and blessings does she learn to bring to others? How does she embody her new understanding and her new gifts?)

Take some time and really savor this creative process.

5. SYNCHRONIZING SOUND FREQUENCY

When you're ready, take 10 minutes for yourself. Close the door. Relax. Read your new story to yourself and really focus on where you feel your new story in your body. Put your hand over this place to help you remember what this level of alignment feels like in your body. When you feel ready, using a good set of headphones, listen to the synchronizing frequency at normal volume and enjoy your personal attunement!

TIME BENDER / MANIFESTING GENERATOR

1. SELF ASSESSMENT AND CONTEMPLATIONS:

Think about your energy. Contemplate whether you feel vital or whether you feel burned out. Take a moment and rank how vital you feel from 0-10

RANK YOURSELF:

0 (BURNED OUT)   10 (VITAL)

RANK YOURSELF ON THE FOLLOWING EMOTIONS:

0 (FRUSTRATION)   10 (SATISFACTION)

0 (REPRESSED)   10 (FREE TO SELF-EXPRESS)

0 (CONFUSED)   10 (CLEAR)

CONTEMPLATIONS:

- How do you feel about being powerful?
- Were you allowed to "follow your flow" as a child?
- Was your power acknowledged and supported by those around you?
- Do you feel comfortable being powerful?
- Is anger a theme in your life?
- Does your fear of anger or your suppression of anger stop you from doing what you want in life?

2. PRIMARY EFT SETUP:

- Even though my frustration keeps me from fully actualizing anything, I deeply and completely love and accept myself.

- Even though I feel disconnected from my natural speed

- Even though I'm frustrated with the manifestations of my life...

- Even though I'm afraid of getting it wrong...

3. QUANTUM QUESTION:

What needs to be healed, released, aligned, and brought to your awareness for you to fully embrace the value of your unique initiating role in the world?

Flower Essence: Quantum Alignment System Time Bender Formula

5. STORYLAB PROMPT:

STORY SPECIMEN: THE MANIFESTING GENERATOR

She was born in a hurry. Even as a baby, she seemed in a hurry to master milestones. As she grew, she explored how much she could do simultaneously. Sometimes, she accomplished a lot. Sometimes, she made a mess of things and had to go back to clean up her mess. Sometimes, it seemed she was skipping from thing to thing.

Her parents and teachers often judged her "mistakes" and her speed. They told her to slow down, and if she focused on one thing at a time instead of "being all over the place," she wouldn't skip important steps or get herself in trouble by "biting off more than she could chew."

She learned to stop trusting her gut and did her best to channel her energy into accomplishing what other people told her she "should" do, eventually drowning out her passion and curiosity. She stopped experimenting and exploring and tried to force herself to stick with one thing, even though her spirit longed for more.

She was often frustrated and angry with the world. It seemed like nothing (and no one) moved fast enough or was as capable as she was, so she often did more than her fair share because it was easier to do it herself than wait for others. She was impatient, had big ideas, and pushed to implement them, even though she often felt that she was pushing against the right timing and the resistance of others.

At work and at home, she carried more than her fair share of the work. Even though this was a way of avoiding the frustration of having to try to get others to go at the same speed as her, she was angry and resentful.

Eventually, she found herself burned out, overwhelmed, cut off from her passion and power, and overcome with the frustration of wanting more...

What comes next in the story? How do you want to write the ending of this story in such a way that it inspires you, lifts you up, and encourages you to continue to reclaim your authentic story in your everyday life?

Do you relate to this specimen? Which parts?

Write your new story starting with the following template:

Once upon a time, there was a _____
_____ (your main character description goes here).

Until one day _____
_____ (What cataclysmic event or experience causes your main character to "wake up" to the true story of who you are? This can be fantastical, realistic, rooted in your real-life experiences or as wild and bold as you choose.)

Until she _____
_____ (What does your main character learn or realize? What lessons and blessings does she learn to bring to others? How does she embody her new understanding and her new gifts?)

Take some time and really savor this creative process.

5. SYNCHRONIZING SOUND FREQUENCY

When you're ready, take 10 minutes for yourself. Close the door. Relax. Read your new story to yourself and really focus on where you feel your new story in your body. Put your hand over this place to help you remember what this level of alignment feels like in your body. When you feel ready, using a good set of headphones, listen to the synchronizing frequency at normal volume and enjoy your personal attunement!

ORCHESTRATOR / PROJECTOR

1. SELF ASSESSMENT AND CONTEMPLATIONS:

Think about your energy. Contemplate whether you feel vital or whether you feel burned out. Take a moment and rank how vital you feel from 0-10

RANK YOURSELF:

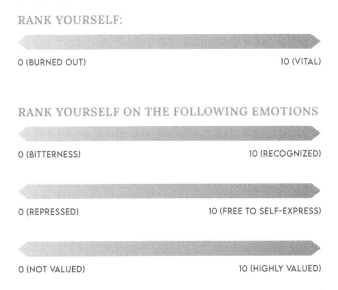

0 (BURNED OUT)   10 (VITAL)

RANK YOURSELF ON THE FOLLOWING EMOTIONS

0 (BITTERNESS)   10 (RECOGNIZED)

0 (REPRESSED)   10 (FREE TO SELF-EXPRESS)

0 (NOT VALUED)   10 (HIGHLY VALUED)

CONTEMPLATIONS:

- Are you bitter? What do you feel resentful about?

- What message do you think your bitterness is giving you?

- Do you value yourself?

- What do you need to heal and release to increase your sense of value and self-worth?

- What is the quality of your spiritual, mental, emotional, and physical energy?

- Do you think you have the energy available for the opportunities you seek?

- What do you need to do to cultivate your energy?

- Do you need to rest?
- Think about some of the greatest invitations you've received in your life.
- How did it feel to be invited or recognized correctly?

2. PRIMARY EFT SETUP:

- Even though I'm exhausted from doing everything, I deeply and completely love and accept myself.
- Even though I don't feel valued, I deeply and completely love and accept myself.
- Even though life feels harder for me than it does for others, I deeply and completely love and accept myself...

3. QUANTUM QUESTION:

What needs to be released, healed, aligned, and brought to my awareness for me to fully embrace the value of my wisdom?

Flower Essences: Quantum Alignment System Orchestrator/Projector Formula

4. STORY LAB PROMPT:

STORY SPECIMEN: THE PROJECTOR

She knew things. Even as a small child, she knew things about people that either astonished them or made them feel very uncomfortable. The truth would spill out of her mouth, and it seemed to her that her profound insights were seemingly common knowledge. Her parents and teachers were often shocked by her boldness and maturity. She was told to keep her insights to herself. She often felt as if her voice and words had no value, even though she knew the things she knew were true and helpful.

She was often accused of being bossy or controlling when playing with other kids. She was left out of the games on the playground because the other kids thought she was weird and different.

Sometimes, the energy of everything around her felt like it was too much, and she would collapse with exhaustion. Her exhaustion often looked like anxiety or overthinking. Sometimes, her body would get sick if she felt overwhelmed.

Her parents would push her to do more, take some initiative, and "put herself out there," but pushing always felt wrong. Despite how wrong it felt, she tried and only exhausted herself more. She felt confused about why things didn't seem to work for her like they did for others. It didn't seem fair that she did all the things she was "supposed" to do with great effort and still didn't have the success that seemed so easy to others.

As she got older, she realized she had insights others didn't have. She knew how to make things better and more efficient. She worked to try to get others to see what she did, but they often didn't hear her or resisted her information. For short bursts of time, she could do more than anyone else. But at the end of the week, this left her feeling depleted and struggling. She was overlooked for promotions and opportunities despite knowing she deserved them. She felt invisible, overworked, and bitter.

Until her body gave out and she crashed...

What comes next in the story? How do you want to write the ending of this story in such a way that it inspires you, lifts you up, and encourages you to continue to reclaim your authentic story in your everyday life?

Do you relate to this specimen? Which parts?

Write your new story starting with the following template:

Once upon a time, there was a _____
_____ (your main character description goes here).

Until one day _____(What cataclysmic event or experience causes your main character to "wake up" to the true story of who you are? This can be fantastical, realistic, rooted in your real-life experiences or as wild and bold as you choose.)

Until she _____
_____ (What does your main character learn or realize? What lessons and blessings does she learn to bring to others? How does she embody her new understanding and her new gifts?)

Take some time and really savor this creative process.

5. SYNCHRONIZING SOUND FREQUENCY

When you're ready, take 10 minutes for yourself. Close the door. Relax. Read your new story to yourself and really focus on where you feel your new story in your body. Put your hand over this place to help you remember what this level of alignment feels like in your body. When you feel ready, using a good set of headphones, listen to the synchronizing frequency at normal volume and enjoy your personal attunement!

CALIBRATOR / REFLECTOR

1. SELF ASSESSMENT AND CONTEMPLATIONS:

Think about your energy. Contemplate whether you feel vital or whether you feel burned out. Take a moment and rank how vital you feel from 0-10

RANK YOURSELF:

0 (BURNED OUT)   10 (VITAL)

RANK YOURSELF ON THE FOLLOWING EMOTIONS

0 (IN LOVE WITH THE POTENTIAL)   10 (RECOGNIZING THE TRUTH)

0 (REPRESSED)   10 (FREE TO SELF-EXPRESS)

0 (DISAPPOINTED)   10 (FULFILLED)

CONTEMPLATIONS:

- Are you disappointed?
- What/who are you disappointed in?
- What needs to be healed, released, aligned, and brought to your awareness for you to recover from disappointment?
- Do you feel responsible for fixing and healing the pain of others?
- Do you need to release yourself from this responsibility?
- Do you feel responsible for helping others meet their potential?
- Do you need to release yourself from this responsibility?
- Are you in the right place? With the right people?
- Do you need to change your environment?
- Are you giving yourself the time you need to make good choices?

- Do you have people in your life who can serve as your sounding board as you talk through your decisions in life?

2. PRIMARY EFT SETUP:

- Even though I'm disappointed in life, I deeply and completely love and accept myself.
- Even though it's hard to reflect on the conditions I experience…
- Even though it's hard to reflect the gap between reality and potential…

3. QUANTUM QUESTION:

What needs to be released, healed, aligned, and brought to my awareness for me to embrace the wonder of the world?

Flower Essences: Quantum Alignment System Calibrator/Reflector Formula

4. STORYLAB PROMPT:

STORY SPECIMEN: THE REFLECTOR

She had big feelings. The energy of the world ricocheted around in her body, making her feel all kinds of emotions. When bad things happened in the world around her, she felt them more than others, and this confused her. Sometimes, the bigness of her emotional expression made her parents struggle. They couldn't understand why everything had to be so emotional. She was often shut down and learned to stifle some of the bigness of what she felt.

She had a big personality and could light up a room. She often had more energy than others, which also led to learning to tone down her personality. She was "too much" for others. She was often told she talked too much, felt too much, and was too intense…

She needed time to make changes. Sometimes, she was pushed and pressured to make changes and transitions before she was ready, which caused her great anxiety. The pressure to adapt quickly often left her scrambling for security, and she often clung to her friendships and significant others in a way that felt clingy and overwhelming. She was sometimes accused of taking all the energy in the room and wanting to be the center of attention, which caused her to shut down her light.

She fell in love with people's potential. She could see the potential in individuals, communities, and even the world. Her ability to see potential made her perspective idealistic and, often, disappointing.

It took her a long time to see whether someone was fulfilling the promise of their potential. She would coach and support her loved ones and friends until the disappointment was overwhelming. It would take her a long time to break these bonds, leaving her depleted and heartbroken.

She had a lifetime of diving "all in" and then trying to figure out how to get out of commitments and promises. She put all her heart and soul into everything and had difficulty setting boundaries and walking away until she couldn't do it anymore...

What comes next in the story? How do you want to write the ending of this story in such a way that it inspires you, lifts you up, and encourages you to continue to reclaim your authentic story in your everyday life?

Do you relate to this specimen? Which parts?

Write your new story starting with the following template:

Once upon a time, there was a _____
(your main character description goes here).

Until one day _____
(What cataclysmic event or experience causes your main character to "wake up" to the true story of who you are? This can be fantastical, realistic, rooted in your real-life experiences or as wild and bold as you choose.)

Until she _____
(What does your main character learn or realize? What lessons and blessings does she learn to bring to others? How does she embody her new understanding and her new gifts?)

Take some time and really savor this creative process.

5. SYNCHRONIZING SOUND FREQUENCY

When you're ready, take 10 minutes for yourself. Close the door. Relax. Read your new story to yourself and really focus on where you feel your new story in your body. Put your hand over this place to help you remember what this level of alignment feels like in your body. When you feel ready, using a good set of headphones, listen to the synchronizing frequency at normal volume and enjoy your personal attunement!

ABOUT THE AUTHOR

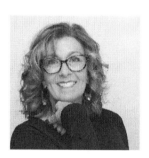

Karen Curry Parker, PhD, is an international Amazon best-selling author of multiple books on personal transformation, spirituality, and Human Design. She is the creator of the Quantum Human Design™ and the Quantum Alignment System™. Speaking, coaching, training, and podcasting on these and other topics for 30+ years, she impacts lives daily worldwide. Her core mission is to help people reconnect with their natural creativity, manifest their desires effectively, and consciously use the frequency of language and narrative to craft a life that best serves themselves and adds more love and joy to the world.

With Quantum Human Design and Quantum Alignment System, she has created certification pathways for new and experienced coaches to add this transformative system to their business practices.

She has featured guests on her award-winning podcast, including Kyle Cease, Gregg Braden, Paul Selig, Dr. Joe Dispenza, and Dr. Gerald (Jerry) Pollack.

Karen is an eloquent speaker, well-versed in many leading-edge subjects regarding humanity's development and future. She teaches audiences engagingly and is adept at employing her sense of gentle humor to increase understanding and retention.

Karen holds a Ph.D. in Integrative Medicine and is working on multiple new books. She is a faculty member at The Shift Network and Omega Institute. Karen has been featured on Bloomberg, Businessweek, CBS, and ABC, as well as various radio shows and telesummits.

Made in the USA
Columbia, SC
02 January 2025

51075694R00062